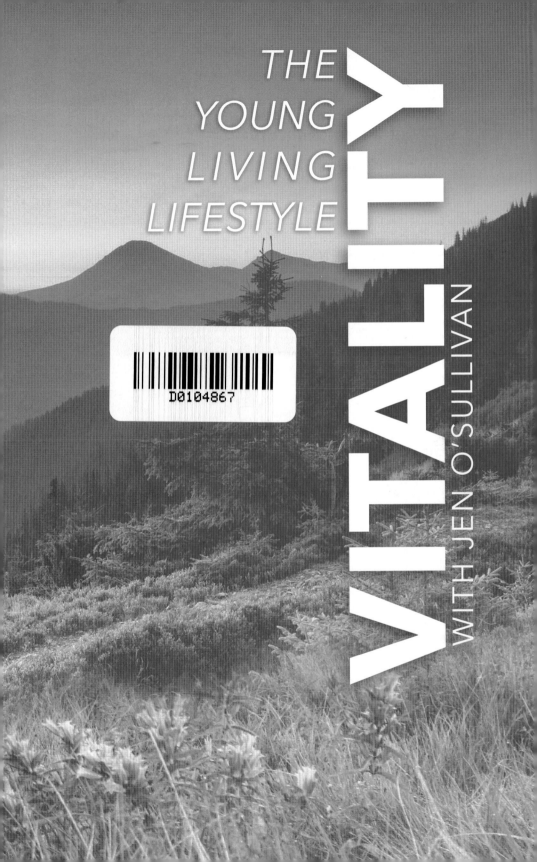

THE
YOUNG
LIVING
LIFESTYLE

VITALITY

WITH JEN O'SULLIVAN

D0104867

# VITALITY: The Young Living Lifestyle by Jen O'Sullivan

Copyright ©2018 by Jen O'Sullivan
www.31oils.com

Book Design by 31 Oils, LLC
Cover Photography by Leonid Tit

ISBN-13: 978-1719596633
ISBN-10: 1719596638

Printed in the United States of America

May 2018

A huge THANK YOU to the following for their help with this project! You all are a blessing to me!

Aleesha Dannielle
Allyson Mobley
Allyson Smith
Amy Cox
Amy Tinker
Ashley Poff
Barb Ferguson
Beth Walters
Beverly Richards
Brie Holst
Carleene Parra
Carmen DeShazer
Caroline Robert
Cathryn Knock
CathyJo Jankens
Christie Hutchinson
Cindy Jennings
Cindy VanFossen
Courtney Byron
Cynthia Edens
Danah Meyers
Deb Brimmer
Denise Klover

Denise Garcia
Gloria-Jean Allison
Jacqueline Ng
Jaime Adams
Janet Bezdziecki
Jennifer Colucci
Joanne Moody
Jonalyn Borja
Judi O'Brien
Kara Shrestha
Kat Atwood
Kimberly DeJesus
Laura Hudnall
Lauren Collins
Leah Vandermeulen
Leslie Borski
Lisa Stoika
Lisa Terranova
Lisa Watt
Lisa Whitener
Margie Duavit
Marianne Wilkins
Mary White

Maryalice Quinn
Melanie Ramsum
Michele Mathiesen
Michele Kovaleski
Michelle Garcia
Monica Campbell
Monika Juliana
Naaznin Pastakia
Nancy LeGrand
Nicole Laeger
Pam VanLoon
Peg Johnson
Peggy Spurk
Sandy Fritsche
Sarah Melissa Lim
Shari Barnard
Sherri Cummings
Stacey Brown
Tamara Snow
Tara Adams
Teri Thompson
Trisha Menzies
Vicki Dunn Cain

The book is humbly dedicated to the hundreds of Young Living members who helped define and shape this book. I am eternally grateful especially to Team Vitality, a group of dedicated Young Living builders who love sharing the beauty of the Young Living lifestyle! What a joy and honor it is to work side-by-side with you on this journey of wellness, purpose, and abundance!

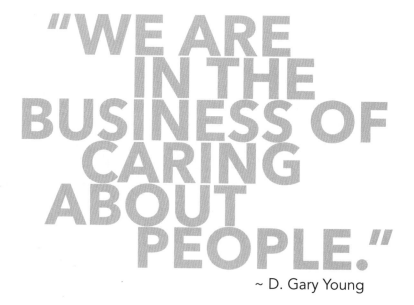

"WE ARE IN THE BUSINESS OF CARING ABOUT PEOPLE."

~ D. Gary Young

# VITALITY

*THE YOUNG LIVING LIFESTYLE*

JEN O'SULLIVAN

# CONTENTS

# "SUCCESS IS LIVING YOUR DEEP BURNING PURPOSE."

~ D. Gary Young

What a blessing and honor it is to be on this wellness journey with you! Making the decision to live a more healthful life is an important step to take. Having the right products and support along the way is crucial. Young Living makes it easy to switch to a more healthy lifestyle because they have done all the research, sourcing, creating, and testing for you!

Young Living is your best partner for a successful lifestyle shift. Young Living produces essential oils distilled from organic plants they cultivate on their own farms. They also create the most bioavailable supplements on the market that utilize essential oil infused whole-food sourced nutrition. They have an amazing personal care product line that contains only sustainable and natural ingredients, including a fully toxic-free makeup line and household cleaning line you will love, plus so much more!

This book is meant to be read one day at a time for the next 30 days. I won't tell anyone if you decide to read it all in one sitting, but get your highlighter pen out and for sure have some sticky notes ready to tag pages. I want this book to look like a rag doll at the end. Reference it and re-read it. Make recipes and share with friends. Most importantly, have fun! I hope this book brings you a life full of health and wellness from the most incredible company on the planet: Young Living.

~ Jen O'Sullivan

**PS: Join the VITALITY Book Club for additional resources on Facebook at www.Facebook.com/groups/VitalityBook**

## DIFFUSER DIRECTIONS

*Directions: Use a cold-water diffuser. Add the essential oils one at a time directly on top of each other in the water or create a synergy, also known as a blend of several oils mixed together. To create a synergy, add them to a clean dropper bottle, then gently swirl the bottle to mix them together and allow them to synergize for 24 hours. Once synergized, add the desired amount of anywhere from 6-12 drops to your diffuser.*

## ROLLER DIRECTIONS

*Directions: Use a 5mL bottle with an AromaGlide fitment. Add the essential oils, then swirl to blend and allow to synergize for 24 hours. Top off with V-6™ oil or the carrier oil of your choice.*

## SERUM DIRECTIONS

*Directions: Use a 5-15mL glass dropper bottle. Add the essential oils, then swirl to blend and allow to synergize for 24 hours. Once fully synergized, top off with the carrier oil of your choice.*

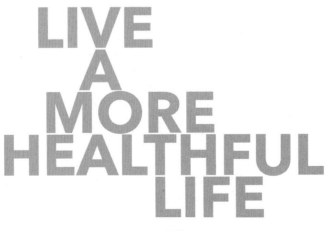

LIVE A MORE HEALTHFUL LIFE

# RECIPES

The essential oil world is fascinating, and once you start down the endless path of health and wellness, you will soon find out the sheer bliss that comes from learning a tried and true recipe that actually works! Time and time again we find ourselves exclaiming, "Wow, that worked!" Even those of us who are well acquainted with essential oils, with many years of experience under our belt, still find limitless joy when we find new recipes and methods to help us support our health and wellness.

Recipes are what everyone wants when they first start out. New people often want exact drop recipes with directions on the exact method and location of application. The first few pages of this book will give you some of the top recipes we all love, and you may find some new ones to try, too!

Not to worry if you are missing an essential oil from a recipe. It is best to leave it out rather than substitute it. If the oil is one of the top two oils listed in the recipe, make sure you get that oil as those are usually the most important. For blends that contain the same amount of drops of each, try to get all essential oils needed for that recipe. All-in-all, don't sweat it! Just have fun and start to play with your oils. They are magic in a bottle, and you will fall in love at first smell!

## TOP 10 DIFFUSER RECIPES

*TOP 10 DIFFUSER RECIPES*

### FRESH AIR
3 drops Peppermint
3 drops Lavender
3 drops Lemon

### SIMPLE DE-STRESSER
3 drops Lavender
3 drops Cedarwood
6 drops Lime

### JUICES FLOWIN'
6 drops Bergamot
4 drops Orange
4 drops Copaiba

### TEA TIME
3 drops Ginger
3 drops Orange
2 drops Cinnamon Bark
2 drops Clove
2 drops Lemon

### RELAX & UNWIND
3 drops Copaiba
3 drops Lavender
3 drops Frankincense

### WORKDAY HUSTLE
5 drops Lemon
3 drops Nutmeg
3 drops Stress Away™

### STUDY SESSION
2 drops Peppermint
2 drops Copaiba
2 drops Lemon
2 drops Frankincense
2 drops Lavender

### HOMEWORK TIME
5 drops Peppermint
3 drops Copaiba
3 drops Lemon

### BURLY MAN
5 drops Bergamot
3 drops Vetiver
3 drops Sacred Sandalwood™

### MID-DAY PICK-ME-UP
5 drops Peppermint
5 drops Lemon
2 drops PanAway®

Get additional diffuser tips in Lesson #6.

*Directions: Use a cold-water diffuser. Add the essential oils one at a time directly on top of each other in the water or create a synergy by adding them to a clean dropper bottle, then swirl to blend and allow to synergize for 24 hours. Once synergized, add the desired amount, 6-12 drops to your diffuser.*

TOP 20 BEDTIME RECIPES

## TOP 20 BEDTIME DIFFUSER RECIPES

3 drops Copaiba
3 drops Frankincense
3 drops Lavender

2 drops Frankincense
2 drops Vetiver
2 drops Lavender
2 drops Cedarwood

3 drops Lavender
3 drops Cedarwood

4 drops Lime
2 drops Lavender
2 drops Cedarwood

3 drops Patchouli
3 drops Ylang Ylang
3 drops Tangerine

4 drops NL Black Spruce™
2 drops Sacred Sandalwood™

2 drops Roman Chamomile
4 drops Lavender
4 drops Cedarwood

3 drops Lavender
3 drops Bergamot
1 drop Valerian

3 drops Marjoram
3 drops Bergamot
3 drops Cedarwood

2 drops Ylang Ylang
2 drops Frankincense
2 drops Bergamot
2 drops Valerian
2 drops Marjoram

BLEND BUMP RECIPES

4 drops Stress Away™
2 drops Frankincense

4 drops Stress Away™
4 drops Lavender

3 drops Stress Away™
2 drops Lavender
2 drops Frankincense
1 drop Vetiver

2 drops Stress Away™
2 drops Copaiba
2 drops Frankincense

3 drops Stress Away™
3 drops Sacred Sandalwood™

4 drops Peace & Calming®
2 drops Tangerine

3 drops Peace & Calming®
2 drops Frankincense
1 drop Vetiver

3 drops Valor®
2 drops Copaiba

4 drops Valor®
2 drops NL Black Spruce™

4 drops Valor®
3 drops Roman Chamomile

TOP 10 SERUM RECIPES

## TOP 10 SERUM RECIPES

### DELUXE FACE SERUM
10 drops Frankincense
10 drops Lavender
10 drops Copaiba

### SACRED 7 FACE SERUM
10 drops Sacred Frankincense™
10 drops Frankincense
10 drops Sacred Sandalwood™
10 drops Myrrh
10 drops Cedarwood
10 drops Hyssop
10 drops Rose

### NO CROW EYE SERUM
15 drops Gentle Baby™
10 drops Myrrh
10 drops Sacred Frankincense™
6 drops Patchouli
2 drops Rose (optional)

### WRINKLE-RELEASE SERUM
10 drops Patchouli
10 drops Sacred Sandalwood™
5 drops Vetiver
5 drops Helichrysum
5 drops Cypress
5 drops Cedarwood

### BLEMISH SERUM
10 drops Tea Tree
10 drops Cedarwood
10 drops Lavender
10 drops Frankincense
10 drops Patchouli
5 drops Blue Tansy

### VAGINAL SERUM
10 drops Tea Tree
5 drops Rosemary
5 drops Lavender

### SCROTUM SERUM
10 drops Tea Tree
5 drops Myrrh
2 drops Peppermint

### CRACKED HEAL SERUM
10 drops Tea Tree
10 drops Lavender
10 drops Frankincense

### UNDERARM SERUM
60 drops Purification®
20 drops Cypress
(top off with Jojoba carrier only)

### BEARD BALM SERUM
9 drops Patchouli
6 drops Bergamot
4 drops Clove
4 drops Rosemary
3 drops Cedarwood
2 drops Lemongrass

### SILKY HAIR SERUM
10 drops Rosemary
10 drops Lavender
10 drops Cedarwood
5 drops Juniper
5 drops Cypress

*Directions: Use a 15mL glass dropper bottle. Add the essential oils, then swirl to blend and allow to synergize for 24 hours. Once fully synergized, top off with the carrier oil.* **Mature Skin:** *Rosehip Seed Oil.* **Blemish Prone:** *Grapeseed Oil.* **Body Application:** *V-6™.* **Vaginal, Scrotum, Beard, and Underarm:** *Jojoba.*

## TOP 10 ROLLER RECIPES

### BREATHE-FREE
6 drops Lavender
6 drops Lemon
6 drops Peppermint

### HAPPY DAYS
5 drops Frankincense
3 drops NL Black Spruce™
3 drops Bergamot
2 drops Lavender
2 drops Lime

### CALM YO' BUTT DOWN
5 drops Vetiver
5 drops NL Black Spruce™
5 drops Sacred Frankincense™
5 drops Lavender
5 drops Cedarwood

### WORK YO BUTT OFF
20 drops Wintergreen
10 drops Clove
10 drops Lemongrass
10 drops Peppermint
5 drops Oregano
5 drops Dorado Azul
5 drops Sage

### ANXI-AWAY
5 drops Sacred Sandalwood™
5 drops Copaiba
3 drops Vetiver
2 drops Lime
1 drop Bergamot
1 drop Lavender
1 drop Sacred Frankincense™

### ON TOP OF THE WORLD
10 drops NL Black Spruce™
5 drops Frankincense
5 drops Blue Tansy

### MIND OVER MATTER
10 drops Rosemary
5 drops Peppermint
5 drops Juniper
3 drops Copaiba
3 drops Lavender
2 drops Frankincense
2 drops Vetiver

### READY FOR BED
10 drops Valerian
10 drops Tangerine
10 drops Bergamot
5 drops Frankincense
5 drops Lavender

### AUNT FLO'S MIX
10 drops Clary Sage
7 drops Marjoram
5 drops Bergamot
5 drops Sacred Frankincense™
5 drops Cedarwood
3 drops Ylang Ylang
2 drops Fennel

### BEARDED BROTHER
8 drops Sacred Sandalwood™
5 drops Bergamot
3 drops Vetiver
2 drops Frankincense
1 drop Lavender

*Directions: Use a 5mL bottle with an AromaGlide fitment. Add the essential oils, then swirl to blend and allow to synergize for 24 hours and then top off with V-6™ oil or the carrier of your choice.*

TOP 10 ROLLER RECIPES

# ADDITIONAL EDUCATION

*Join the VITALITY Book Club for additional resources at*
*www.Facebook.com/groups/VitalityBook*
*Sign up for the eCourse at www.31oils.com/oils101*
*Apps: "The EO Bar" and "Live Well with Young Living"*
*Connect on Facebook: The Human Body and Essential Oils group*
*Shareable Facebook Content: www.Facebook.com/JenOSullivanAuthor*
*Instagram: @JenAuthor*
*Printed Resources: www.31oils.com*

# BOOKS TO CONSIDER

*The Essential Oil Truth, The Facts Without the Hype*
*French Aromatherapy, Essential Oil Recipes and Usage Guide*
*Essential Oil Make & Takes*
*Essentially Driven, Young Living Essential Oils Business Handbook*
*Live Well (the PSK educational mini book)*

# THE VITALITY LIFE COMMITMENT

*I _____ am full of health, wellness, and life.*
*I choose to live my life with an abundance of vitality!*
*Signed:*

*_____ Date _____*

**VITALITY: The Young Living Lifestyle** *by Jen O'Sullivan*

You are about to embark upon an incredible wellness journey through the full Young Living product line! The largest portion is on essential oils since that is our foundation. This book is full of information for both new and seasoned oilers. The lessons in this book will help you to get the fullest grasp on Young Living and how to completely reset your healthy lifestyle. This is a commitment to health and wellness that your mind, body, and soul will thank you for. I hope this book becomes a trusted friend in your education of the true essence, beauty, and magic of essential oils and Young Living!

This book will help you to live a more full and vitality-filled life. Start now with a simple, yet very important personal commitment to your health. Take a moment to write out a healthy lifestyle statement below, then sign and date it. Share it with the world to give yourself greater accountability. Take a photo of it, post it on Facebook or Instagram and use the hashtag #ChooseVitality then tag me, too! I am honored and blessed to be a part of your journey!

Let's do this together! We can have a more vitality-filled life today. Let's become the best version of ourselves so we can accomplish our purpose in this world! Are you ready? I most certainly am! Here we go!

## LESSON #1
# *THE PREMIUM STARTER KIT*

Congratulations on taking your first step towards a more vitality-filled life with Young Living! You should have your Premium Starter Kit and are now ready to dive into the amazing world of essential oils. If you don't have a PSK (Premium Starter Kit) from Young Living, what are you waiting for? It is by far the best way to get started using essential oils. Young Living has put together the top 11 oils that everyone needs along with an incredible diffuser and several fun samples. At over 50% off it is a no-brainer! Connect with the person who shared this book with you or, if you don't have an oily friend to help you, feel free to reach out to me personally. I would be honored to welcome you to the Young Living family!

# *HOW TO BECOME A MEMBER*

Purity is key when choosing the right essential oil company. The right person to assist you on your journey is also important. My goal is to help you learn the best way to use your essential oils, and to share more ways to add health and wellness to your family and home. There are several ways you and your friends can get started.

Becoming a member with Young Living has some great perks!
- 24% off retail prices
- 50% off the retail price of the PSK with membership.
- No additional fees, your kit purchase is your membership fee.
- No mandatory minimum monthly orders.
- Order what you want, when you want.
- Access to Essential Rewards to get up to an additional 25% back on your monthly order.
- Access to a community of health-conscious people who want to share this journey with you!

The moment you buy your Premium Starter Kit you are eligible to get a paycheck from Young Living with a commission of $50-$100 per person that signs up using your member number! Think of 5 friends who may want to share in this oily journey with you, share this book with them or plug them into one of the many online education groups so you can experiment together!

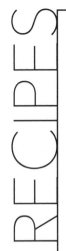

# THE PSK SINGLES

LAVENDER (single species)
- Usage: Topical and Aromatic
- Good for: Emotions, Calming, Mental Focus, Skin Health, Hair Health

*also available in:*

LAVENDER VITALITY™ (single species)
- Usage: Internal
- Good for: Respiratory, Immunity, Digestive, Nervous, Limbic, Endocrine, Hormones

FRANKINCENSE (single species)
- Usage: Topical and Aromatic
- Good for: Skin Smoothing, Calming, Emotions, Positivity, Mental Clarity

*also available in:*

FRANKINCENSE VITALITY™ (single species)
- Usage: Internal
- Good for: Immunity, Limbic, Endocrine, Respiratory, Throat, Nervous, Circulatory

COPAIBA VITALITY™ (single species)
- Usage: Internal
- Good for: Calming, Nervous, Circulatory, Respiratory, Muscles

*also available in:*

COPAIBA (single species)
- Usage: Topical and Aromatic
- Good for: Calming, Focus, Emotions, Skin Smoothing, Muscle Soothing, Clarity

LEMON VITALITY™ (single species)
- Usage: Internal
- Good for: Circulatory, Renal, Respiratory, Digestive, Immunity

*also available in:*

LEMON (single species)
- Usage: Topical and Aromatic
- Good for: Cleansing, Uplifting, Mental Clarity, Brightening, Emotions

PEPPERMINT VITALITY™ (single species)
- Usage: Internal
- Good for: Respiratory, Circulatory, Digestive, Flushing, Appetite, Hypothalamus, Energy

*also available in:*

PEPPERMINT (single species)
- Usage: Topical and Aromatic
- Good for: Mental Clarity, Focus, Stimulating, Post Exercise, Soothing, Cooling, Relieving, Purifying

## USAGE IDEAS

Essential oils have hundreds of uses per oil! Below are a handful of ideas to get you started. To learn about all the other uses, join our educational groups online or feel free to ask!

- Frankincense: Add one drop daily to the nape of your neck for better mental clarity.

- Lavender: Add 6 drops to your cold-water diffuser before bedtime to help relax.

- Peppermint: Apply one drop to your hand, cup over nose, and breathe deeply for an invigorating experience.

- Lemon: Add one drop to your water for a refreshing experience.

- Copaiba: Apply one drop to the back of the neck for better focus.

21

# THE PSK BLENDS

Blends (aka synergies) are a great way to get added benefits from essential oils. These are some of the most beloved synergies of all time. Many companies try to make copycat versions, but fail to hit the mark.

THIEVES VITALITY™ (multi-species)
- Ingredients: Clove, Lemon, Cinnamon bark, Eucalyptus, Rosemary
- Usage: Internal
- Good for: Immunity, Purifying

*also available in:*
THIEVES® (multi-species)
- Ingredients: Clove, Lemon, Cinnamon bark, Eucalyptus, Rosemary
- Usage: Topical and Aromatic
- Good for: Health, Strengthening, Mouth Health, Ear health, Purifying

DIGIZE VITALITY™ (multi-species)
- Ingredients: Tarragon, Ginger, Peppermint, Juniper, Fennel, Lemongrass, Anise, Patchouli
- Usage: Internal
- Good for: Digestive, Flushing

*also available in:*
DIGIZE™ (multi-species)
- Ingredients: Tarragon, Ginger, Peppermint, Juniper, Fennel, Lemongrass, Anise, Patchouli
- Usage: Topical and Aromatic
- Good for: Calming

RAVEN™ (multi-species)
- Ingredients: Ravintsara, Lemon, Wintergreen, Peppermint, Eucalyptus Radiata
- Usage: Topical and Aromatic
- Good for: Health, Opening, Calming, Relaxing, Flushing, Uplifting, Cooling

CITRUS FRESH™ (multi-species)
- Ingredients: Orange, Tangerine, Grapefruit, Lemon, Mandarin, Spearmint
- Usage: Topical and Aromatic
- Good for: Cleansing, Purifying, Uplifting, Calming, Energizing

*also available in:*
CITRUS FRESH VITALITY™ (multi-species)
- Ingredients: Orange, Tangerine, Grapefruit, Lemon, Mandarin, Spearmint
- Usage: Internal
- Good for: Circulatory, Renal, Respiratory, Digestive, Immunity, Metabolism

PANAWAY® (multi-species)
- Ingredients: Wintergreen, Helichrysum, Clove, Peppermint
- Usage: Topical and Aromatic
- Good for: Soothing, Stimulating, Post Exercise, Regenerative, Energizing, Cooling

STRESS AWAY™ (multi-species)
- Ingredients: Copaiba, Lime, Cedarwood, Ocotea, Vanilla, Lavender
- Usage: Topical and Aromatic
- Good for: Calming, Focus, Relaxing, Emotions, Grounding, Mental Clarity

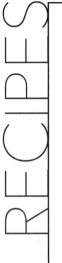

# THE DIFFUSERS

The Premium Starter Kit comes with your choice of top-notch diffusers.

**The Desert Mist Diffuser** – The Desert Mist diffuser has a stylish modern design and is perfect for any room. It is an atomizer, humidifier, and aroma diffuser in one easy-to-use product. It features up to 10 hours of run-time depending on the mode you use. It has 11 different light settings including a candle-like flickering mode.

**Dewdrop™ Diffuser** – This workhorse diffuser is also a family favorite. It is the only silent diffuser and features 4 hours of run-time with automatic shut-off. It is an atomizer and humidifier all in one.

*The Dewdrop or the Desert Mist comes standard in the PSK or you may upgrade to one of the following:*

**The Aria™ Ultrasonic Diffuser** – The Aria™ has a gorgeous glass dome with a solid American maple wood base. This diffuser comes complete with multiple settings from 1-3 hours, a range of LED color options, plus it plays relaxing spa-inspired music or you may plug in your own personal music device. It's an ultrasonic atomizer and humidifier all in one.

**The Rainstone™ Diffuser** – This stylish black high-end clay base ultrasonic atomizer and humidifying diffuser comes with multiple settings including timer from 1-8 hours, LED control with various color options, as well as the ability to turn on or off the ionizer.

## USAGE IDEAS

- Thieves®: Add 6 drops to your cold-water diffuser during the day.

- PanAway®: Apply one drop to shoulders and lower back after a workout.

- Raven™: Rub one drop over chest and neck for a soothing experience.

- DiGize™: Rub one drop over abdomen or in a capsule as needed.

- Citrus Fresh™: Add a few drops to your diffuser for a bright smelling room.

- Stress Away™: Apply 1-2 drops on wrists during the day every 4 hours.

## LESSON #2

# *THE ESSENCE OF ESSENTIAL OILS*

Essential oils changed my life in 2007 and I know they are about to change yours! Seriously, these little bottles have become my "gems". I cannot WAIT to share with you all the information that is packed into my overstuffed brain, so I am going to attempt to do it a bit at a time, piece by piece. Each daily lesson will contain 3-6 areas for you to digest. That's it.

Sprinkled along the way I will give you some of my favorite recipes to try. If you are wanting more information right away, check out The EO Bar app. It has so many recipes and education topics your head will spin! In all cases, if you have any questions, let me know. Consider me your personal "Oil Lady" through the pages of this book because I want you to enjoy the oily fun as much as I do. Let's get started!

# *WHAT ARE ESSENTIAL OILS?*

Essential oils are nature's purest essence of the botanical they are pulled from. The "oil" is extracted primarily through steam distillation or cold pressing. They are often called the "life-force" of the plant. They help the plant to regulate itself and add health and overall wellness. Essential oils can work in much the same way for us.

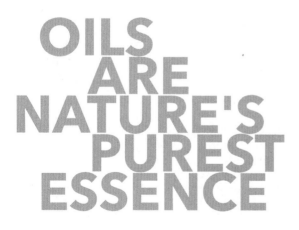

OILS ARE NATURE'S PUREST ESSENCE

## CARRIER OILS

Carrier oils help dilute an essential oil, and are great for spicy or hot oils or to use as bases for lotions and serums. There are dozens of carriers and it is a good idea to try a few to find out which ones you like. Look for organic, cold pressed, pure, and unrefined carrier oils. Some of the most common carrier oils to start out with are:

- V-6™ Vegetable Oil Complex
- Fractionated Coconut
- Grapeseed
- Coconut
- Sweet Almond
- Rosehip Seed
- Jojoba

## TOXINS IN OUR HOMES

Most personal care products contain some of the worst toxic chemicals. The National Institute of Occupational Safety and Health (NIOSH) conducted a study that tested the toxicity of 2,938 chemicals. NIOSH found that 884 are toxic, 778 cause acute toxicity, 376 are skin and eye irritants, 314 may cause biological mutations, 218 may cause reproductive complications, and 146 may cause tumors. Source: United States House of Representatives Report from the National Institute of Occupational Safety and Health (NIOSH), 1989.

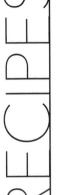

**RECIPES**

TOPICAL

Take care of tired muscles and joints by rubbing on one drop of PanAway™ with carrier oil.

INFUSED WATER

Add 1-2 drops of Lemon Vitality™ to your glass or stainless steel water bottle, fill with cold water then drink to help flush your system.

DIFFUSER

In your cold-water diffuser add 3 drops each of Lavender, Lemon, and Peppermint for one of the most loved diffuser blends known to mankind!

TRY THIS!

Add a drop of Peppermint to your hand, cup over your nose and breathe deeply. Rub the rest on the back of your neck with carrier oil for a pick me up!

## LESSON #3

# HOW TO USE ESSENTIAL OILS

What do you do? Drink the stuff? Put it in your tea? Snort it? OK, so really...I know, I know, sometimes we may feel like total lame ducks trying to navigate through it all, so here are some short lessons on how to use them and some safety tips.

### AROMATIC

This is the most common use of essential oils because they are essentially aromatic. You can simply open a bottle and take a deep breath and you will get great benefits. You can also rub them on your hands, cup your hands over your nose, and breathe deeply. Another, more popular way, is to use them in your cold-water diffuser.

### TOPICAL

Essential oils may be used all over the body. Some body parts are more sensitive than others, so make sure to use a carrier oil. Place a drop into your palm and rub the essential oil on the back of the neck, bottom of the feet, wrists, spine, top of the head, or anywhere there is a need.

### INTERNAL

Only use pure essential oils that are labeled for consumption from the Young Living Vitality™ line. You may add a drop or two into an empty capsule and top off with a carrier oil, use a drop under your tongue, add a drop to a glass or stainless steel water bottle, or add a drop to honey or another edible item. More advanced use would be to create suppositories (rectal) or pessaries (vaginal).

### SAFETY FAQS

Essential oils are potent gifts from nature that can often be more powerful than expected. In order to prevent misuse of these precious oils and ensure their maximum benefit, Young Living has created a very helpful safety and usage guide. Read up on all their great tips and most commonly asked questions at: www.youngliving.com/en_US/discover/essential-oil-safety/

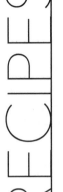

# GENERAL SAFETY

- A carrier oil helps dilute an essential oil.
- The term "neat" means to use without a carrier oil.
- A "hot" oil is one that feels warm. Use a carrier oil.
- If you get essential oils in your eye, rinse with milk, rice milk, or carrier oil. Do not flush with water.
- Do not apply a citrus oil to the skin if you are going in the sun. Wait 12-18 hours.
- Always dilute with carrier oil if under age 12.
- If you experience an uncomfortable response, add carrier oil or discontinue use.

# HOT OILS

Some oils can feel quite hot when applied. They won't actually burn you, but man-oh-man, they can feel like an inferno, especially if you get them in your eyes and you try to flush them out with water. If any get in your eyes, simply flush it out with cold milk (plant or animal based milk work well).

For your skin, if you apply an essential oil and it feels uncomfortable or your skin gets red, simply add more carrier oil or lotion to calm the area. Lip balm works great too in a pinch!

## TOPICAL

Remember the diffuser recipe from Lesson 1? I want you to get the same three oils: Lavender, Lemon, and Peppermint. Put one drop of each into the palm of your hand, add a drop of carrier, blend with your finger, and then rub it on your skull just behind your ears and down your jawline on both sides. You can thank me later!

## INFUSED WATER

Add 2 drops of Lemon Vitality™ and 1 drop of Peppermint Vitality™ to your glass water bottle. Give it a little shake before each sip.

## LESSON #4

# SIMPLE TIPS TO GET STARTED RIGHT

We've learned a lot so far but let's back up just a bit so we can go over it more. The best thing you can do is re-read your notes and then re-watch a few videos or check out some additional content. Are you figuring it out? Are you becoming an oil addict like me? Be careful, it can get VERY addictive! When something works and you can see the benefits right away it is hard not to get excited. You are well on your way to taking back your health!

I remember when I got my first set of oils. Seriously, it was like Christmas morning. I didn't know where to start. It is almost too simple. Just open them up, smell them, put them on your body, anywhere... just get started. So, here are a few simple tips to start you out.

- Keep your oils out of direct sunlight.
- Keep them all upright so they don't leak.
- Keep lids hand tight but do not over tighten.
- Share them with friends! They will love you for it!
- Have oils in your purse, at your desk, bedside table, vanity, kitchen counter, everywhere and anywhere!

# DETOX AND SYSTEM FLUSHING

So many people want to detox their body of the toxins they have been exposed to. They have figured out that over the years they have built up something, they may not know exactly what, but they know it MUST be detoxified. They will go on full body cleanses, colon cleanses, fasts, pills, all sorts of things. Before you do any of that, it is super important to figure out specifically what you need to detoxify. Essential oils are amazing at helping to flush out your body. Check out "The EO Bar" app and look under "System Flushing" for some really great ways to flush out your system. A wonderful way to get started is to start drinking 1-2 drops each of Peppermint and Lemon Vitality™ oils in your water every day for 7 days, then take a break for a couple days, and start again!

## CHOOSING A BRAND

By now you probably have heard about several other essential oil companies and may be wondering, did you get the right oils company? I am right there with you! I have tested 22 essential oil brands to date. Just so you know, there are hundreds upon hundreds of essential oil companies and with so many popping up every year, it is impossible to keep track. Oils are popular and just because someone is great at marketing doesn't mean they are the best. Buyer beware!

Based on all my research and side-by-side testing, Young Living is by far the best. My testing conclusions are based on the pure, authentic aroma (I knew they were not pure if I got a synthetic headache from smelling them during testing) and their breadth and depth of action. These two are the most important in my quest for pure, medicinal-grade essential oils. So far, no one has even come close to Young Living. If you are not currently using Young Living oils, I encourage you to test those oils side-by-side with Young Living. You will be surprised!

## RECIPES

### DIFFUSER

Add 3 drops Frankincense and 2 drops Lavender to your cold water diffuser before bedtime for a relaxing, calming aroma.

### INFUSED WATER

Play with citrus oils! Add 1-2 drops of 3 or 4 of the following from the Vitality™ line: Orange, Tangerine, Jade Lemon, Grapefruit, Lime, and Lemon. Add 1 drop of Peppermint or Spearmint Vitality™ for an extra pop!

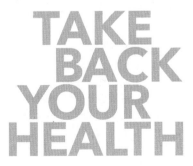

TAKE BACK YOUR HEALTH

# HOW TO SIDE-BY-SIDE TEST FOR PURITY

One of the simplest ways to test oils against each other is to buy as close to the same oil as possible. Look for the correct Latin binomial. Rather than Lavender or French Lavender or True Lavender, look on the label for the botanical that is actually in the bottle: *Lavandula angustifolia*. Use the 5 methods below to test your oils.

Buy three oils directly from each company such as Lavender, Lemon, and Peppermint. You may choose a different set of oils, as long as you already know their specific action and how they work on you personally.

### FREEZE TEST
Once your three test bottles arrive, place them on their sides, unopened, in your home freezer. Check after 24 hours to see if any froze. These three oils should not freeze prior to opening. Let them thaw to room temperature.

### AROMA TEST
Smell them each from the bottle. Note the top note aroma. Drip a drop into your hand, rub your hands gently together and inhale deeply. Note the aroma. Do you get any headache from the smell? Does it smell sweet? Does it smell like it came from the earth and like the botanical it came from? What does it smell like after 30-60 minutes on your skin? Note all of these things. Give several hours between each species and use one hand for one company and one for the other. Example: Lavender from Company A on your left hand and Lavender from Company B on your right.

### SYNERGY TEST
Get two brand new dropper bottles in 5 or 10mL size. Put 10 drops of each oil from one brand into one dropper and 10 drops of each oil from the other brand in the other dropper. Place the cap on the dropper and swirl around. Let this sit for 24 hours. After 24 hours, take one drop from each and do the aroma test from #2 above. The blend you created should smell fresh. If it smells off, you know for sure there are synthetics in the oils.

# IN-HOME TESTS.

## *BREADTH OF ACTION TEST*
Using a little carrier oil, drip two drops into your palm and use your finger from your other hand to rub the blend on your skull, behind your ears and down your jawline on both sides. Note the action within 30 seconds. Sit down and rub a little of the blend, with carrier oil, on your cheeks next to your nose. Close your eyes. Note the sensation you feel. Is it a harsh feeling, cutting feeling, deep cleansing feeling? Wait several minutes before opening your eyes or adding more carrier oil. Be careful not to get any in your eyes.

## *FILLER TEST*
Get a piece of Cotton Rag paper (not copy paper) and a pencil. Create a large graph with two rows of three boxes (six boxes total). Label the upper left corner of each box with the company name and the oil used. Drip one drop from each oil into the correct box. Keep paper on a glass or ceramic table (do not place on plastic or wood, it will contaminate the test). Check back in 30 minutes. If any of the oils are completely gone without a stain, they use alcohol as a filler. Good oils should still show a wet mark. Check back after 12 hours. Only the Lemon should leave a faint yellow tint. If the tint is green or some other color for the Lemon, that is not a good sign. If either of the other oils, Lavender or Peppermint, show a ring or mark on the paper (hold it up to the light to check as well) then they are using a carrier oil as a filler.

# LESSON #5
## *QUALITY*

Right about now your brain is either seriously overloaded or starving for more! Let's go with starving. I like to call it "The Oil Epiphany Effect." You "get it" now you want to "get it" even more. Isn't it fun finding out about something you never knew you should know? So, here we go...get ready to get your learning cap on.

## *THE FOUR TYPES OF ESSENTIAL OILS*

There are four types of oils on the market today. Most of the ones labeled "pure essential oils" or even "therapeutic grade" fall into the manipulated or augmented category because it is a very common practice to remove heavier "earthier" smelling molecules for a more pleasing aroma.

### *AUTHENTIC*
100% pure (Single species and multiple species labeled as a blend)
Authentic essential oils are 100% pure throughout the bottle. There are no added synthetics or other species of oils unless they are labeled as a blend or synergy and are using only authentic essential oils in that blend. They make up the small minority of all essential oils on the market.

### *MANIPULATED OR AUGMENTED*
100% pure (Blends labeled as Singles, Fractionated, or Rectified)
Perfumers are often hired by essential oil companies to help make the final product smell more pleasing and less earthy. They will take away some of the heavier molecules (fractional distillation) or add very small amounts of another species to enhance the aroma or to make it match a previous batch aroma (rectification).

### *PERFUME*
Pure with synthetic
You will often see an essential oil labeled as "pure" when they are not. There is a percentage of pure essential oil and a percentage of synthetic to enhance the final aroma. These types of oils often cause headaches and do not have any therapeutic action.

### *SYNTHETIC*
100% Synthetic
These "essential oils" are not essential oils at all. Because there are no labeling regulations on the term "essential oil," full synthetic oils are able to be labeled as pure and sold to unsuspecting consumers to increase profit. These often smell nothing like the original plant, but they can be very close, and that is why a consumer may not know they are synthetic and have possible severe negative reactions.

# AUTHENTICITY

If you are wondering, Young Living singles are all authentic. The oils they use in their blends are also authentic. Very few companies use truly authentic oils. Let's take a brief look at what Seed-to-Seal® means. I encourage you to visit the website too. It is also a fun experience for little ones!

### STEP 1: SEED

Seeds are carefully selected by experts based on the previous year's crop potency and effectiveness. No other company can guarantee the proper seed selection.

### STEP 2: CULTIVATE

Using only sustainable methods, Young Living's farming practices set the bar around the world. They use above organic grade standards.

### STEP 3: DISTILL

Young Living is the largest innovator of oil distillation using several proprietary techniques. These techniques are copied by competitors but never duplicated.

### STEP 4: TEST

Young Living tests all oils using internal labs, and third party testing. Their standards are higher than international standards. They use up to 20 tests on each batch in triplicate two separate times during the process.

### STEP 5: SEAL

Each bottle is carefully packaged to ensure a perfect product shipped directly to you. You never have to worry about your oils being adulterated from third party resellers.

RECIPES

## DIFFUSER

To calm even the busiest of households and office spaces.

- 6 drops Bergamot
- 4 drops Orange
- 4 drops Copaiba

## TOPICAL

If PanAway® is the workhorse of tension oils, Deep Relief Roll-On™ is the racehorse. Roll this bad-boy all over the tips of your fingers, then liberally rub your entire scalp. Do this 2-3 times. This will help your head be happy again!

# PURITY MATTERS

There are two major modifications that the majority of essential oil companies practice so they are able to provide essential oils to the general public that will be more acceptable to their customers. These oils, while more pleasing to the general public, would be considered less than authentic essential oils. The two types of modifications are fractional distillation and rectification. Both of these modification practices are common with every essential oil company on the market today. It is your job to determine if the company you use practices these modifications.

# RECTIFICATION (RECTIFIED ESSENTIAL OILS)

Rectification is a correction that is made when a batch of essential oil smells different than the previous batches. This is often the case with natural products because of variations in growing conditions such as rain, sunshine, temperature, soil conditions, and harvesting conditions. You would not expect every single apple you eat to taste the same. Because we get used to a particular aroma, if it is coming out of a product in a bottle, we expect it to smell the same as the last bottle. When a bottle comes to us that smells different, we call customer service to get our money back as something must be wrong with this batch.

The truth is, each essential oil batch should smell different. Slight variations to even more pronounced variations should be common. Since the industry knows the general public will not like these variations, almost all companies practice rectification. Rectification is when they add in molecules from another species or from a synthetic in small amounts to make it match not only the gas chromatography mass spectrometry report, but also to match the aroma from the previous batches for consistency. These additions are impossible to detect on a certificate of analysis report and even the most trained eye can miss the addition of synthetics or other species present in the batch. It is why organoleptic testing is a very important part of the batch test process.

# FRACTIONAL DISTILLATION (FRACTIONATED ESSENTIAL OILS)

One of the most common and widespread practices in the Aromatherapy industry in the United States of America is the "fractional distillation" of essential oils, also called fractionated essential oils. Americans are known to want everything smelling fragrant. They love their candles, scented plug-ins, and car air fresheners. The age of science that bombarded us in the 1950's is wreaking havoc on us all today in the form of synthetic headaches and hormone issues. But Americans still love their scented fragrance and may not realize it may be the source of their headaches and hormone issues. Due to this market trend, the aromatherapy industry thinks you, the consumer, would rather have a better smelling essential oil over therapeutic value.

When you smell an essential oil that has gone through the process of "fractional distillation" you get a much more pleasing aroma from the oil. Here is how fractional distillation works. The distillery processes the plant material through their distillation stills. The end product is a pure, unadulterated, true botanical essential oil. It smells like the actual plant does. After the original processing of the plant material, either the original distillery or often times the buying company, will take the raw oil and fractionally distill the oil 1-3 times to take out the heavier, dirtier smelling (earthier) molecules.

The best way to visualize this is to consider coconut oil. You can buy raw coconut oil that is solid and opaque at room temperature. If you get fractionated coconut oil, it is clear and liquid at room temperature. This is exactly the same concept applied to essential oils. Those two carrier oils are not the same, nor are essential oils that have been fractionated the same either. Fractionated essential oils may smell better, but they do not have the same therapeutic action. In the case of coconut oil, fractionated is fine to use, but knowledge is power, so it is best to understand that in some cases using fractionated coconut oil is more beneficial in the case of rollerballs, but the raw form is better if you are using it to clean the makeup off your face.

A fractionated essential oil, while still considered pure, is something completely different. It will still have therapeutic qualities, but those qualities will not have an action that is as deep, or that lasts as long as its true botanical un-fractionated counterpart. When a company decides to remove the heavier molecules, they are removing the earthier aroma, but they are also removing the very nature of the oil's ability to stay on and in your body longer, and they are removing a part of the synergy of the molecules that make them work best together. Fractionated essential oils are altered. They are not the true botanical, and are lower quality.

How can you know if your company does this? The answer is quite simple. Smell them. Bring a few of your oils to a garden nursery such as your Lavender, Lemon, Peppermint, and Spearmint. If you have Melissa ask for Lemon Balm and if you have Helichrysum ask for Curry. For Lavender, check the species your company sells and ask for that species. Most of you will have *Lavandula angustifolia*. Peppermint is hard to find, so ask specifically for it. Most better nurseries will carry it. For Lemon, you can use the rind of a lemon from the grocery store and scratch the surface with your finger to get the essential oils to release.

Once you find the plants, open your bottle, drip a drop into your left hand, then gently crush some of the leaves between your fingers of your right hand and smell your right hand fingers against your left hand palm. If the oil in your left hand palm smells sweeter, you have a fractionated oil.

Young Living is one of a very few companies that does not use fractionated essential oils. All of their direct competitors use fractional distillation and it's obvious through a simple organoleptic smell test. D. Gary Young, the founder of Young Living Essential Oils®, was far more concerned with giving his customers the true pure botanical than hoping his customers would love the smell. Young Living oils smell earthy in most cases. Some of you would rather stick to your fractionated essential oils because you are using them for mild application and a desire to make your living areas smell more pleasing. I applaud you for removing your toxic candles and plug in scented items. It is a huge step toward health and wellness.

Each company is different and will not disclose if it fractionates or rectifies. It is important for you to understand these two modification methods and decide for yourself if you are desiring to use unaltered essential oils from the botanical source, or altered essentials oil that will placate your need for consistency.

# STEWARDSHIP IN PURITY

We all grew up smelling something "like" lavender, but not actual lavender in most cases. Synthetic lavender is in everything from soaps and lotions, to shampoo and even lingerie drawer lavender bud filled sachets infused with synthetic fragrance to make the aroma last longer! World-renowned Aromatherapist, Dr. Kurt Schnaubelt states the following in his book "Healing Intelligence of Essential Oil: The Science of Advanced Aromatherapy"

> *"French export data shows that 250 tons of so-called Fine Lavender are exported annually. The statistics of the Association of Lavender Growers in Volx show that less than 20 tons are in fact distilled. Ironically, this glaring fraud is obvious to those who can read the gas chromatograms, ostensibly recorded to demonstrate purity. Generally neither local vendor nor customer can read the chromatogram, but both associate proof of authenticity with its sheer existence. In reality most Lavender chromatograms passed around in the marketplace prove adulteration."*

Did you know the term "essential oil" doesn't have any definition other than "fragrance". Popular and well known perfume companies could start stating that their fragrances use only pure essential oils and the labeling agencies would be perfectly fine with it, even though 100% of the bottle uses synthetic. There are no labeling regulations, no purity regulations, and no one policing any of the essential oils on the market. Basically any company can create anything they want, using synthetic toxic chemicals and slap a label on it stating it is pure and organic. If you have a few minutes, take time to watch this video about what goes into our personal care products: https://youtu.be/pfq000AF1i8

Young Living produces 100% pure, fine, unrectified, unadulterated, unfractionated, essential oils. They own 15 farms on 5 continents and is growing each year. To keep up with the growing demand, Young Living has 3 pillars of purity sourcing: Corporate Farms, Partner Farms, and Seed-to-Seal® Certified Suppliers. Young Living controls everything from the seeds used to the final production. No company can claim to have the amount of farms and control that Young Living has over purity. When it comes to their Seed-to-Seal® Certified Suppliers, Young Living only works with farms that are fully trained in the stringent quality of Seed-to-Seal®. They undergo audits and screenings and all oils are tested using 15-20 tests in triplicate two times during the process: once when they receive it and once just before bottling. Read the following section to learn about all the tests.

# PURITY TESTS

There are 20 tests that should be considered by any essential oil company, unfortunately most only do 4-7. Young Living tests every batch of essential oil using up to 20 different tests, in triplicate, two different times during the production process. If the batch makes it through all of the tests during the first phase, then it goes to bottling, where it is tested again with all of the tests in triplicate. Some oils are tested using 15 or more tests, as some oils do not need certain tests. The testing is very thorough. It takes 20 people just over a week to perform the required testing on each batch to determine if it meets Young Living's standards. Some oils get a total of 120 total tests. Here is a list of all the tests they perform.

1. **Gas Chromatography-Mass Spectrometry (GC-MS):** GC is the method of separating the individual molecular compounds in a substance that can be vaporized without being damaged. MS is the means by which the final detected molecular compounds are analyzed.
2. **Gas Chromatography-Flame Ionization Detector (GC-FID):** This may be added to the GC-MS and is a means to detect if there are any non-organic materials.
3. **Viscometry:** Measures the thickness of an oil.
4. **Densitometry:** How light or dark an essential oil is when light passes through.
5. **Specific Gravity:** This compares the density of water to the density of an essential oil to obtain a purity measurement.
6. **Refractometry (Refractive Index):** How an essential oil bends light based on its molecular structure.
7. **Polarimetry:** How an essential oil bends polarized light based on its molecular structure. Uses Optical Rotation.
8. **Inductively Couple Plasma (ICP-MS):** Measures metals in an essential oil. It can detect one bad molecule in a billion good molecules. This is like finding one drop of bad water in an Olympic-size pool!
9. **Inductively Coupled Plasma-Atomic Optical Emission (ICP-OES):** Measures metals in the oil using light.
10. **High Performance Liquid Chromatography (HPLC):** Similar to the GC-MS, but uses pressure instead of heat like the GC-MS.
11. **Fourier Transform Infrared (FT-IR):** Measures the chemical bonds within the compounds.

# TWENTY TESTS

12. **Automated Micro-Enumeration:** Counts the good and bad bacteria. (Microbiological Test)
13. **Disintegration:** The rate at which an oil disintegrates.
14. **pH:** The specific pH of an essential oil.
15. **Flashpoint:** Specific flashpoint of the oil and safety test. The lowest point of temperature when an oil vaporizes into a gas and then can be ignited with an external fire source.
16. **Microscopy Analysis**: Broad range of data obtained to analyze the molecular structure of each oil from particle identification to molecule size.
17. **Combustibility:** The point at which an oil catches fire using oxidation without the addition of fire.
18. **Chiral Chromatography:** Separates optical isomers. Optical isomers are mirror images (racemic) like your hands. When compounds are synthesized in a lab, we almost always get a racemic mixture. This shows if the oil is pure or synthetic. Man-made products have two peaks that are the same, pure (natural) products have one.
19. **Isotope Ratio Mass Spectrometry (IR-MS):** Helps to monitor and detect the presence of synthetics. This is based on the atomic mass and is often called Carbon Isotope Ratio Analysis. It measures ratios of isotopes (atom with a different weight). Such as a Carbon mass of 12, 13, or 14 depending on the added neutrons. The oils need to be the exact mass to the atmosphere to ensure purity. Young Living is the only company in the USA that owns this machine and they have two of them!
20. **Organoleptic Testing:** A sensory method of subjective testing where a scientist looks at the oil for optical purity and smells the oil for purity. This is done by very experienced people with a mental library of essential oil aromas and sometimes tastes. This type of testing will usually also be done by physical action to test the oil's therapeutic response within the body.

## LESSON #6

# DIFFUSING BENEFITS

Cold-water diffusers are essential to any family that wants to promote a more healthful environment.

The benefits of diffusing:
- Supports a more restful sleep
- Supports better daytime focus
- Promotes healthy air quality
- Helps force dust to the floor
- Creates a healthy ionized room
- Creates an uplifting environment
- Helps neutralize odors
- Safer alternative to candles
- Helps to elevate moods
- Promotes better energy

# DIFFUSER TIPS

### TYPE OF DIFFUSER
Check to see if you are using a cold-water diffuser or an atomizer. Cold-water diffusers are most common today. Atomizers use oils without dilution and should only be used for a maximum of around 10-15 minutes. Cold-water diffusers may be used for up to eight hours when used properly.

### AMOUNT OF ESSENTIAL OIL
If using a cold-water diffuser, check your water well size. Most 4 hour diffusers have a 100-200mL water fill-line capacity. You only need to use 4-6 drops per 100mL of water, or 2-3 drops per hour of run time.

### CREATE BLENDS FIRST
Make sure you consider synergizing essential oil singles together first to create blends before adding them to your diffuser. Using single essential oils one at a time is fine, but it will produce different results as the water will encapsulate single oils as you add them to the water.

### USE BLENDS ALONE
Try not to use multiple blends together in your diffuser. You are welcome to do so, however pre-determined blends are specifically designed to have a wonderful synergistic effect and when you add other synergies it creates something possibly too diluted to work as intended. You may use blends with other single essential oils. This is called "bumping" a blend.

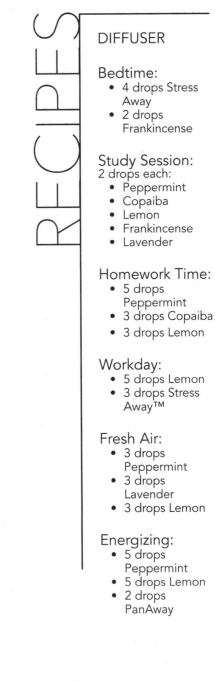

## CLEAN ONCE A WEEK
Make sure to give your diffuser a good cleaning at least once a week. It is recommended that you clean it after each use. Use a little rubbing alcohol and a sponge or the scrub brush that came with your diffuser.

## SURFACE PLACEMENT
Place your diffuser on a hard flat surface. It is best to put it on a location that is not made out of organic material such as wood. If you use a mat, make sure it is not too thick as this could impose on the air vent and your diffuser may not work properly.

## ROOM SIZE
Try to match the correct diffuser for the size of your room. Most 100-200mL diffusers work great for a standard size 100-150 square foot sized room. Larger output diffusers, such as the Aria™, are for larger spaces, such as a living room.

## PETS
Make sure your pets have another space they can retreat to if they do not want to be around the diffuser. Do not use diffusers in an area where your pets are trapped. Use citrus oils and oils high in terpenes and phenols with caution around dogs and cats.

## INFANTS
The use of a diffuser with infants can help calm your baby and is a wonderful way to introduce oils to the nursery. Use one drop per hour of cold-water diffusion for up to four hours.

### DIFFUSER

Bedtime:
- 4 drops Stress Away
- 2 drops Frankincense

Study Session:
2 drops each:
- Peppermint
- Copaiba
- Lemon
- Frankincense
- Lavender

Homework Time:
- 5 drops Peppermint
- 3 drops Copaiba
- 3 drops Lemon

Workday:
- 5 drops Lemon
- 3 drops Stress Away™

Fresh Air:
- 3 drops Peppermint
- 3 drops Lavender
- 3 drops Lemon

Energizing:
- 5 drops Peppermint
- 5 drops Lemon
- 2 drops PanAway

# CLEANING YOUR DIFFUSER

Keep your Young Living diffuser working at its optimal performance by cleaning after each use. Simply pour out any remaining liquid after use, rinse with water, then add some rubbing alcohol. Use the scrubbing wand or a sponge, clean all areas where oils were present. Rinse with fresh water, pour out and let dry or fill up to use again. It's best to clean between uses or at a minimum once a week. Make sure you do not get water in the air intake hole. If you get water in the air intake hole by mistake, turn the diffuser upside down to shake out excess water then let dry for 24 hours before use. For hard to clean areas in the Rainstone™ Diffuser it is best to buy a baby bottle scrub brush with long handle.

You may use a half capful of Thieves® Household Cleaner for optional cleaning if you do not want to use the recommended Rubbing Alcohol. This will not void your warranty.

# DIFFUSING DURING PREGNANCY

Using oils aromatically in a cold-water diffuser with 2-3 drops per hour of diffusion is recommended. Diffusing in a cold-water diffuser is the mildest form of essential oil use and is very beneficial during pregnancy, labor, and delivery. Steer clear of the "do not use" list below as singles. The following list should also be avoided for use with babies:

- Clary Sage
- Idaho Tansy (Blue Tansy is safe)
- Hyssop
- Fennel
- Sage
- Wintergreen

# BEDTIME RECIPES

### SLEEP SUPPORT COLD-WATER DIFFUSER RECIPES:

You may play around with pre-mixed synergies by bumping them with 1-2 drops of a single essential oil that is not contained in that synergy. An example would be Peace & Calming II™ with Cedarwood. Many people choose to bump a pre-mixed synergy with an oil contained in that synergy such as Stress Away™ with Lavender. Finding the right combo for you is the key. We are all different and your body will respond to a mix that is just right for you. The most effective and easy way to use essential oils is in pre-mixed blends. Try 4-6 drops of any pre-mixed calming synergy such as Stress Away™, Peace & Calming®, Peace & Calming II™, Gentle Baby®, or Valor®. See several customer favorite diffuser recipes to the right.

# DIFFUSE FOR HEALTH

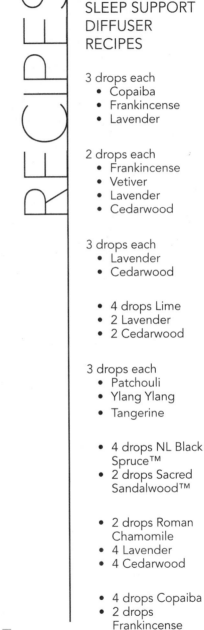

SLEEP SUPPORT DIFFUSER RECIPES

3 drops each
- Copaiba
- Frankincense
- Lavender

2 drops each
- Frankincense
- Vetiver
- Lavender
- Cedarwood

3 drops each
- Lavender
- Cedarwood

- 4 drops Lime
- 2 Lavender
- 2 Cedarwood

3 drops each
- Patchouli
- Ylang Ylang
- Tangerine

- 4 drops NL Black Spruce™
- 2 drops Sacred Sandalwood™

- 2 drops Roman Chamomile
- 4 Lavender
- 4 Cedarwood

- 4 drops Copaiba
- 2 drops Frankincense
- 2 drops Stress Away™

## LESSON #7
# *HOSTING A PARTY*

Are you enjoying your love affair with your oils? Aren't they a blessing? Take a moment to consider sharing what you have found with others. When I find something that works and it blesses me, I want to share that joy with others. A super easy way is by hosting a Make & Take party. This book will help you get an idea for what to do, but if you want to dig deeper, pick up the book "Essential Oil Make & Takes" on Amazon.

HOSTING TIPS
- Invite a few of your friends.
- Make it low key. Nothing too fancy.
- Don't have a bunch of food. Make it duplicatable!
- Pick only one recipe to make rather than multiples.
- Keep the item under $5.
- Get the book "Essential Oil Make & Takes" for more helpful tips.

# *LAVENDER*

Lavender is one of the most widely used fragrances in the world, and according to the Association of Lavender Growers in Volx, France, 90% of all Lavender essential oil is synthetic. You will get zero therapeutic action from synthetic Lavender. Young Living's is the purest you can get. When you use pure Young Living Lavender Vitality™ internally it can support cardiovascular, immune, respiratory, and nervous systems. Lavender is also one of the most well-known and well-loved essential oils. It is commonly referred to as the "Swiss Army Knife" of oils.

Studies have shown that diffusing Lavender while taking tests, improves test scores! SCORE! Add Lavender to your diffuser during homework and study hours, then arm your student with a diffuser bracelet or necklace to smell while taking a test. Here are a couple fun recipes using Lavender:

- Add a few drops of Lavender to your daily face cream and serum. Apply morning and night for a soothing and calming experience.
- Add 1-2 drops Lavender Vitality™ to a pitcher of lemonade for an amazing spa drink. You can thank me later!

## WHAT IS SUBLINGUAL?

Sublingual means to place something under your tongue. Putting a drop of essential oil under your tongue, such as Frankincense or Digize Vitality™, helps the oil bypass your digestive system and go directly into your circulatory system. It is a great way to use oils! TIP: once you drip the oil under your tongue do not move your mouth for 30 seconds. Keep it closed and still. You will be surprised that the oil will not be spicy, nor will it have much taste if you let it absorb without moving your tongue. Drip one drop of the following from the Vitality™ Line under your tongue as needed: Frankincense, DiGize™, Thieves®, or Copaiba.

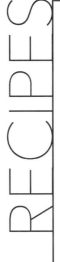

RECIPES

### DELUXE FACE SERUM

The Deluxe Face Serum is bliss in a bottle... and you don't even need to buy a bunch more oils to make it. Get a 15mL glass dropper bottle. Buy your favorite carrier oil. I recommend organic pure Rosehip seed oil or Grapeseed oil. Drip 10 drops of Frankincense, 10 drops of Lavender, and 10 drops of Copaiba into the bottle and swirl to blend. Then top off with carrier oil and swirl again to blend. Rub this on morning and night. No need to use your chemical-laden face creams any longer, this is all you need! So get on it... make that serum!

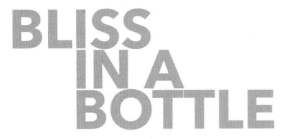

BLISS IN A BOTTLE

# WHEN YOU CRAVE OR HATE AN OIL

There are two types of specific responses to oils. This is not your normal or average response, but when you have an INTENSE response to the smell. This would not be an actual physical reaction, but an emotional response. You either seriously hate it or seriously adore it. With each response there are two potential things at play: your limbic system or your physical body. Let's start with the love response.

When you open a bottle and love love love it, there are usually two responses you will have. The "curl-up-in-a-ball-on-a-comfy-couch-and-smell-the-oil-for-hours" response or the "I-don't-know-why-but-I-kind-of-feel-like-I-want-to-eat-this-oil" response. The first one is based on the limbic system remembering a time in your life that was amazing or abundant with love that becomes a core memory blanketed in a wonderful smell. It is why so many love Stress Away for it's sweet vanilla aroma. It brings us back to our childhood days of making cookies with mom or grandma.

The second response is based on your physical need of the oil. Anytime you smell an oil that you feel like you could eat you love it so much, like PanAway®, that would mean your physical body is craving it. You may have just finished an intense workout and your body says, "YES!!! GIVE ME THAT NOW!" Again, please remember, these are only intense love responses to oils. You LOVE it and your limbic (memory) system kicks in, or you LOVE it and your physical body kicks in saying you need it now.

Now onto the "hate" response.

Yes, "hate" is a strong word, but it is fitting in this instance. A strong dislike does not count. I don't like most floral aromas because that is a personal preference, not an intense response. The word "hate" would not count here. If you smell an oil and hate it, as in you are repulsed by it or want to run from the room, it means one of two things: your body is telling you no, do not use it, or your body is telling you, yes, you need it. The trick is figuring out which one it means. Your body has a built-in smell reactor to things that are bad for you or your body does not need. Such is the case for rotten milk or rancid meat. When you smell those things you have a gut response and you instinctively know you need to avoid it. That is the same here with oils. A good example is when you are pregnant and smell an oil that you used to love but now can't stand. Simply don't use it until your body tells you it is OK again through smelling it periodically.

The second reason is a bit more interesting. When you smell an oil and want to run from the room and you get an intense angry feeling from it, like you want to smash the bottle or can't put your finger on it, but it just makes you mad, that is your limbic system at work. This means you need it emotionally. Something happened to you that this oil will help.

I find it best to start by applying it to the bottom of my feet every day for 30 days. Then smell it again. This oil will burrow into the crevices of your body to help release whatever this negative emotional response is reacting to. Sometimes it will dawn on you why that smell was so disturbing to you, like a memory from a traumatic experience that had that smell.

Often we see this trauma response with Geranium or the oil Joy™ because of parents divorcing or some personal trauma in the 70s or 80s. That was a very popular fragrance back then (Geranium) so if anything bad or traumatic happened to you in the 70s and 80s this would be the case for you. Use the oil, over and over again until you can clear the tucked away trauma.

Broken down to its simplest form:

- INTENSE LOVE/DESIRE = Limbic (fond memories and will help with emotions)
- INTENSE LOVE/CRAVING = Physical Body (somewhere in your body you need this oil to support health)
- INTENSE HATRED/DISGUST = Don't use the oil. Trust your gut.
- INTENSE HATRED/ANGER = Your Emotional Body needs this oil so use it!

# LESSON #8

# *EXPANDING YOUR KNOWLEDGE*

I was terrible in my science classes in high school. Nothing made sense to me. Then I got heavily into essential oils. I wanted to know why and how they worked the way they did. In life I experienced how incredible they are but I wanted to know more. This lesson will help you dig a little deeper. If you want to dive into 48 mini lessons that are really easy to understand, I encourage you to get "The Essential Oil Truth" on Amazon or head over to www.31oils.com to get the book pack. But let's start with a few fun things you may not know!

## *THE ORIFICE REDUCER*
The orifice reducer is the milky plastic part at the top of the essential oil bottle that allows one drop to come out. It is best not to touch this with your fingers as oils from your hands and skin cells will get into your oil and over time will cause oxidation. Don't worry if you have been touching them, but you may want to try to remember it is best not to touch. Instead drip one drop over your hand or desired location or in a water bottle.

## *NUMBER OF DROPS*
There are 85-100 drops per 5mL bottle and 250-300 drops per 15mL bottle. Why the difference? It depends on the oil's viscosity, or how thin or thick it is.

## *TEMPERATURE*
Oils are perfectly safe to ship in extreme temperatures. Both hot and cold. It is best not to store oils in a hot area, but if they are left out in the shipping box and it is super hot all day, not to worry. Simply allow the bottles to fully cool to room temperature before opening. If you open an oil while it is hot, the lighter constituents, namely the monoterpenes, will escape right out of the bottle.

## RESTFUL SLEEP

Does sleep elude you? Essential oils do not help you actually sleep, they work in conjunction with your endocrine system to help support each excretion. For example, diffusing a calming oil such as Stress Away™ or Peace & Calming® during the day works with your cortisol excretions and helps you focus. When used at night when your body is producing melatonin and your cortisol has worn off, it will help your mind calm down and focus and then your body is more ready to fall asleep. Fascinating!

A favorite night time diffuser recipe is to add 2-3 drops each of Frankincense, Vetiver, Lavender, and Cedarwood. This would be great in the morning too when you are just starting your day for better focus!

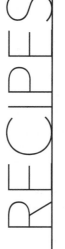

INTERNAL

One fun recipe in the book "French Aromatherapy" that has people always wondering about the name is "The Crazy Lady." It has 1 drop Endoflex Vitality™ with 3 drops Orange Vitality™. Add those to the bottom of your water bottle then add your water. The name? Well, honestly when my hormones are a little crazy, I become a little crazy... just a little. So, The Crazy Lady is a great way to help support your crazy hormones!

# EMPOWERING KNOWLEDGE

## LESSON #9

# *CONSUMING ESSENTIAL OILS*

Consuming essential oils has long been debated in the aromatherapy world. Most aromatherapists will tell you it is absolutely not safe. They are correct on some level. Most essential oils on the market are not safe to consume simply because they are laced with synthetics to make them smell better and to make them cheaper to produce. The reality is, if you have a fully pure essential oil that is processed correctly, and is from a species that is consumable such as Lemon, Peppermint, Lavender, then yes, it is safe to consume. It is important to know some basics, but know that hundreds of thousands of people have been consuming essential oils for centuries without any issues at all. If you would like to understand more about why consuming essential oils is so controversial, read more in the book "French Aromatherapy".

# *VITALITY™ VS. REGULAR*

The FDA (Food and Drug Administration) helps consumers know what they are getting. Safe and accurate labeling is important. Young Living is one of the only essential oil companies in the world to have a dedicated line of consumable essential oils. Their consumable product line is called the Vitality™ line. The oil inside the bottle is exactly the same as the regular bottle. There is no difference in the oils inside the bottle other than the label.

Why is there a need for two different labels on exactly the same product? Consumer might get confused if their vitamin C was labeled for consumption AND topical use. So...do I crush it up and spread it on my skin? Ha! While most of us understand that an essential oil can be used for aromatic, topical, and internal purposes, the FDA wants us to comply by making a distinction on the labels. Any other company that labels their oils as all three uses is outside of FDA regulations and could be subject to huge fines! Young Living stands behind honoring safe labeling practices and you can rest assured that any oil in the Vitality™ line is safe to consume. Any oil that is in the larger 15mL bottle, and is also in the Vitality™ line bottle, with the same name, is also safe to consume.

# LIVE WITH VITALITY

## DISPERSING OILS

"Friends let friends drink essential oils!" You are my friends and I would not steer you wrong! A common argument is that essential oils could burn the mucous membrane of your esophagus as you drink a drop in water. This is sort of true if you are using a spicy oil such as Cinnamon Bark or even Peppermint. Something to consider is using a dispersant. I personally will add just a smidgen of sea salt to my water bottle, then drip the oils in, then add the water. I like to use Pink Himalayan because of the micro minerals. The oils grab onto the salt and it helps disperse it. Give it a little shake before you take a sip and don't add too much salt. The salt is also healthy for you in this very small amount.

## OIL & WATER

Oil and water don't mix. This idea is correct, but flawed. Oily oils and water don't mix. Essential oils do have molecules that will sit on the surface of water, but if you place a metal straw in a glass of water, then drip one drop of Lemon Vitality™ or Peppermint Vitality™ on top, wait 10-15 minutes, and take a sip, you will notice the flavor is all the way at the bottom. Why? Simple. Essential oil molecules are both extraordinarily small (under 300 atomic mass units) and are extremely volatile (they want to move). So try this one yourself and you will see!

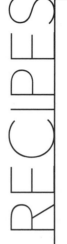

RECIPES

### SMOOTHIE

Using Slique® Shake Mix or Pure Protein Complete™, follow the directions on the label to make the shake and add some frozen berries and 3 drops of Orange Vitality™ or Tangerine Vitality™. One of my faves is using the chocolate Pure Protein Complete™ mix with Tangerine Vitality™. So yummy! For a more creamy shake put in 1/4 cup Greek yogurt.

### INFUSED H2O

I love Tangerine Vitality™ in my water. It is the sweetest tasting essential oil and is so refreshing. Simply drip 1-3 drops into your water and you will love it!

## LESSON #10
# *EXPLORING PHEROMONES*

The way your body smells at the skin level is like a pheromone. Basically it is a secretion or excretion of hormones that have a scent. They attract or repel the same species. It is why my man smells amazing to me, but probably not so much to you.

Essential oils are the pheromones of the plant and insect world. They sometimes attract as in the case of Lemongrass and bees, or they repel as in the case of Lemongrass and mosquitoes. There are several ways to use essential oils to our advantage with both our own species and others. Let's dive in!

# *STINKY FEET*

I love the outdoors. I am always gardening, walking, hiking, cycling, or mountain biking. With being outdoors, come lots of critters. I don't mind most of them, but the mosquitoes tend to LOVE me. I am a total mosquito magnet. Well, about 6 years ago my husband declared he had enough of my stinky feet. I bashfully went into my office to research what to do about stinky feet. It turns out Tea Tree is a great oil to use that helps with foot odor.

I looked at my stash and was out of Tea Tree so I grabbed Purification® which contains Tea Tree. I tried it...and it WORKED! Literally all day long in my shoes with my feet armed with one drop of Purification® on the bottom. But guess what else happened!? Every time I used Purification® on the bottom of my feet, which was every day from that day forward, I noticed something amazing! NO MORE MOSQUITO BITES! Say WHAHHHT??? Read up on the next section to understand why it worked.

## THE 20 MINUTE RULE

Our bodies are smart! When you drip a drop of essential oil such as Purification® on the bottom of your feet, in 20 minutes your skin will have a certain scent only noticeable to certain insects that will not be pleasurable to them. Some insects, however may be attracted to you, so make sure you know which ones to use for which types of outings.

Why does this work? There are around 100 trillion cells in our bodies, and one drop of essential oil contains over 40 million trillion molecules! It takes 20 minutes for an essential oil to reach every cell in your body from the time you apply them. This means every single cell in our body, in 20 minutes, is covered by 400,000 essential oil molecules!

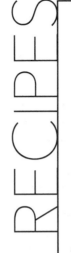

RECIPES

TOPICAL

Purification® is the oil most commonly used to freshen stinky feet. One drop on the bottom of the feet in the morning gets the job done. It is also a mom favorite for their school-age kids to help keep critters away.

DIFFUSER

Change the mood in the room before your spouse gets home. Run your diffuser with the following blend and then turn it off the diffuser 30 minutes before they enter the home. Let the romance begin!

- 5 drops Orange
- 3 drops Joy®

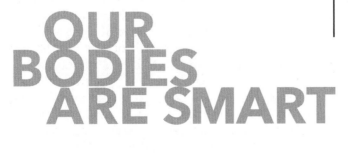

OUR BODIES ARE SMART

**LESSON #11**

# *ESSENTIAL OILS AND EMOTIONS*

Our emotions are driven by several elements, including our environment, what we consume, our body chemistry, and hormones. There is no "one-size-fits-all" approach when it comes to essential oils, so it is important to try several before you give up. This lesson will teach you some of the important ideas and concepts to remember when using essential oils to help support our emotions.

Take Stress Away™ for example. Stress Away™ is a favorite blend of many Young Living fans, and it's commonly joked that users would bathe in it if they could. It contains a small amount of Vanilla absolute, making it a favorite among kids and adults alike. Children often call it their "vanilla ice cream oil". This blend contains 5 single oils: Copaiba, Lime, Cedarwood, Ocotea, and Lavender with a touch of Vanilla absolute. When you use it, the aroma and the therapeutic action instantly calm you. It helps you focus during the day and calm down at night.

## *JOY & TRAUMA*

Joy tends to escape us most days. Too much to do, and not enough time to do it. We get caught up in the daily grind. The essential oil Joy™ was created with a synergy of oils such as Bergamot, Ylang Ylang, Geranium and others. The floral citrusy aroma helps our cells to feel full and happy. Interestingly, it often has the opposite effect on the user. Feelings of rage or sadness may pop up instead! Our limbic system is very sophisticated. It remembers things we do not. It places smells as tags for memories. Geranium was used in a popular fragrance in the 1980s. Those who have a strong dislike to this oil often went through a trauma with their mother in the 80s. Possibly a divorce or a mom who was overworked that took it out on you. It's life. The interesting thing is if you really do not like this oil and you had some trauma in the 80s, it may be your body telling you it wants to heal. I encourage you to think back to the time of trauma and release those emotions. Use Joy™ on your heart or on your feet if you really dislike the smell. Do this several times a week for as long as it takes to see emotional healing begin to happen. Guess what? Once you release those angry feelings, you will actually enjoy the smell of Joy™!

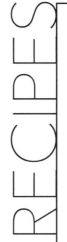

# LIVING ANXIOUSLY

Living day in and day out riddled with worry, fear, and anxious feelings sets us on a course to damage our adrenals. Not only does it completely derail our life, but it will give you long term endocrine damage if you are not careful. Getting your stress and anxious feelings lowered is important. You may consider taking CortiStop® to help support healthy cortisol production. Essential oils are also wonderful to help calm and relax us when we are feeling out of control. Here is a great on-the-go recipe.

Using a 5mL rollerball add:
- 5 drops Sacred Sandalwood™
- 5 drops Copaiba
- 3 drops Vetiver
- 2 drops Lime
- 1 drop Bergamot
- 1 drop Lavender
- 1 drop Sacred Frankincense™

Place all essential oils in the bottle and swirl to blend. Then top off with V-6™, fractionated coconut oil, or your favorite organic carrier oil. Use this on your wrists and front and back of neck as needed throughout the day. Smell the aroma on your wrists too!

# SADNESS

Sadness is a real thing. We don't want to be sad, but sometimes it just hits us like a wave or a ton of bricks. Try blending the following in your hand and rubbing it on your chest and back of neck, then cup your hands and breathe in deeply.

- 1 drop Bergamot
- 1 drop Frankincense
- 1 drop Vetiver

## DIFFUSER

Our emotions surrounding our loved ones can, at times, be volatile. A great way to add some harmony and balance into your home is to diffuse Orange essential oil. It also gets our juices flowing and will help open up your libido. Try rubbing a few drops on your pulse points too!

## TOPICAL

Release™ is an essential oil known to help balance and release emotions. A great way to use it is to drip a drop into your palm, rub hands together, take a deep breath, then rub the rest all over the back of your neck! Sweet release!

## LESSON #12

# *ESSENTIAL OILS AND OUR HEAD*

Our head is an interesting thing. Think about it for a sec. It is the viewpoint from which we live. We see, hear, taste, smell, and touch with our head. We think, create, reason, learn, laugh, love, anger, understand, and cry. The list goes on and on. Head health is paramount to our overall health. Did you know you can support your entire head with essential oils? Of course you did! Let's dig in once again!

The blood-brain barrier is in place so nothing can get in. It is a wall of tight junctions around all the capillaries (blood vessels) protecting all the cells inside the brain. God designed it so well that He knew man would mess things up with synthetics so He made sure nothing could get into it that was made by man. His medicine, essential oils, on the other hand gets right in! Essential oil molecules have an atomic mass unit (amu) of under 300. They have estimated that in order to break the blood brain barrier a molecule needs to be around 500 amu. Drugs are larger than that and cannot break through.

The next time you are wanting to focus on head health, grab your favorite essential oil and anoint yourself. Try one of the following: Drip a drop of Northern Lights Black Spruce™ directly on the top of your head. Rub some Frankincense or Copaiba on the back of your neck. Dip your thumb into some Lavender and hold it to the roof of your mouth for 15 seconds. Drip a drop of Sandalwood on your hand, rub together, cup over your nose, and take as deep and as long of a breath as you can. Your head will be happy!

# *FOCUS SUPPORT: COPAIBA VS. CBD OIL*

Our mind tends to wander and have squirrel moments just about every other minute. We often feel out of control and sometimes at dis-ease. Copaiba to the rescue! Copaiba, pronounced kō-pī-bah or kō-pī-ee-bah, is steam distilled from the oleoresin, which is a mixture of the essential oil and resin of the plant. It is excellent to help calm and soothe muscles and joints. Young Living states, "Known for its gentle, woodsy aroma, Copaiba essential oil is a product of steam distilling the gum resin tapped from the Brazilian Copaifera reticulata tree. With high levels of beta-caryophyllene and a uniquely sweet aromatic profile, Copaiba oil helps create a relaxing atmosphere when diffused or applied topically."

Copaiba has high levels of beta-caryophyllene. While Young Living cannot state an oil does this or that from a medicinal or even therapeutic standpoint, they do give you very, very important crumbs that are more important than you might think. Any time you see them call out a seemingly chemistry type term, go ahead and look that up on Google. Notice anything interesting? Cannabis contains around 30% caryophyllene (aka beta-caryophyllene). Copaiba contains upwards of 40-70%! The question always gets asked if Copaiba and CBD are the same and can you substitute Copaiba for CBD.

The simple answer is, no. Copaiba is very different from CBD oil. There are similar properties but they are not to be swapped. When we make recipes it is important to note that one part of an oil does not make the whole of it. For example, an apple is not just Vitamin C but a whole host of vitamins and nutrients. Over 10,000 phytochemicals have been estimated to be in just one apple. Copaiba is helpful in two very important ways: to make a path for other oils to get in more readily and to help our minds calm and focus.

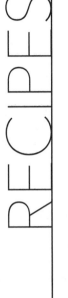

## RECIPES

### DIFFUSER

Enjoy lazy afternoons with this diffuser recipe.

- 5 drops Lemon Myrtle
- 1 drop Blue Tansy

### TOPICAL

Place one drop of Copaiba on the back of the neck and one drop of your favorite Spruce on the top of your head for better mental clarity and focus.

## Common Uses
- Internal with Vitality – Supports cardiovascular, nervous, and respiratory systems.
- Topical and Aromatic – Helpful to calm and focus the mind when diffused or applied topically. Helps to soothe muscle tension.

## Best Practices
- Internal with Vitality – Add a drop to a capsule to support healthful body systems.
- Topical – Apply after strenuous exercise. Rub a drop on the back of the neck and temples to support cognitive function.

# SACRED FRANKINCENSE™ VS. FRANKINCENSE

"Sacred Frankincense™ essential oil comes from the distillation of the resin of the Boswellia sacra frankincense tree. This oil is ideal for those who wish to take their spiritual journey and meditation experiences to a higher level." ~ Young Living

Alright, so what is the REAL skinny?

Most companies do not have true Sacred Frankincense™. In fact, some carry a trio or quad of Frankincense oils and some even label it as just Frankincense hoping consumers will not notice it is a blend and not a single species! A quick peek at a competitor's website and you will note that their Frankincense is labeled under "Single Oils" yet the ingredients list "Resin from Boswellia carterii, sacra, papyrifera, and frereana". That is four different tree species altogether! That is definitely not a single oil!

I'd like you to do a little research now. Go ahead and look up the constituent makeup for both Frankincense (*Boswellia carterii*) and Sacred Frankincense™ (*Boswellia sacra*) essential oils. It will blow you away to see how very different they are. So when a friend gives you a recipe that calls for Sacred Frankincense™, and you only have Frankincense, realistically you should not sub out the oils. They are different and do different things for us. It is fun to start seeing how they differ. Generally, Frankincense (Boswellia carterii) is the one to use for your skin and for calming, while Sacred Frankincense™ should be used for greater mental clarity and a heightened spiritual awareness.

### MONOTERPENES: ALPHA-PINENES
Very bioavailable and rapidly metabolizes.
- Sacred Frankincense™ (*Boswellia sacra*) 53-90%
- Frankincense (*Boswellia carterii*) 30-65%

### L-LIMONENE (CHIRAL OR MIRROR IMAGE TO D-LIMONENE)
Skin support
- Frankincense (*Boswellia carterii*) 8-20%
- Sacred Frankincense™ (Boswellia sacra) 2-7.5 %

### SESQUITERPENES BETA-CARYOPHYLLENE
Calming molecules
- Only found in Frankincense (*Boswellia carterii*) 1-5%

## AROMA HEADACHES

I get headaches from pretty much any and all synthetic aromas and smells. I don't get headaches from food or plant aromas. Anytime I go into a mall it is like a war zone for me. Dodging stores left and right. From perfumes to candles, headache bombs are everywhere. So what gives? The majority of our headaches to various aromas come from synthetic fragrances, not the real thing. So when a friend comes over and says they cannot stand strong smelling things I ask them, "Do you run when someone peels an orange?" They always say, "No." I tell them essential oils are the same exact thing. Young Living essential oils are so pure that it is exactly like peeling an orange. I have the person imagine that I have an orange, then open the bottle of Orange EO and they smile. It is that simple! Get rid of the candles and synthetic fragrances and say hello to Mother Earth. God got it right! All other brands are cheap impostors.

## EYE HEALTH

Take care of your eyes by adding some Lavender and Frankincense to your nightly eye cream. I create a serum with a 15mL bottle of carrier oil and 10 drops each of Lavender and Frankincense. After I clean my face and eyes, I drip 2-3 drops of this serum in my hands and gently rub around my eyes. It is mild enough not to upset your eyes so feel free to apply liberally all over, even the eyelashes!

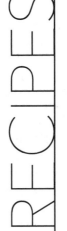

**RECIPES**

TOPICAL

Happy Blend: Using a 5mL roller bottle, create a synergy using

- 5 drops Sacred Frankincense™
- 3 drops NL Black Spruce™
- 3 drops Bergamot
- 2 drops Lavender
- 2 drops Lime

Swirl the bottle to synergize the essential oils and then top the bottle off with grapeseed oil. Place rollerball top on. Swirl the bottle to blend all ingredients. Roll on the bottom of your feet focusing on the pads of your big toes, on your wrists, and back of the neck 2-4 times per day or as needed. Put a little in your hand, cup your hands over your nose and breathe in deeply three times. For a sweeter fruitier blend do 3 drops each Lime and Lavender.

## LESSON #13
# *RAINDROP® TECHNIQUE*

The Raindrop® Technique is thoroughly loved by anyone who has experienced it. It is a method of massage along with the use of several essential oils along the back area. This method of essential oil application was developed and taught by Gary Young back in the late 80s before Young Living was an official company. There are many versions and adaptations of this technique and I will do my best to teach you in one lesson how to do it the way it was intended. While variations are perfectly fine, getting one the way Gary developed it is absolutely incredible. I hope you get a chance to get one or learn with a friend and give each other a session. You will love it!

A fun thing to do is measure the height of the receiver prior to the application and then again afterward. Our spine is riddled with things we would rather not have hanging out there and sometimes causes unwanted compression. Post-raindrop you will find those unwanted items have been flushed and the receiver can stand taller. Note: this does not always happen but it is fun to see it when it does.

# *RAINDROP® BY GARY YOUNG*

The following link shows the original version as taught by Gary Young. See the videos below. Note, he gives his original recipe for Valor! Woohoo!
GARY'S ORIGINAL VIDEOS: www.tinyurl.com/ycx8tbfc

# *THE KIT*

The Raindrop® Technique Kit is the perfect way to get started. It comes with all the oils and a couple massage oils to compliment the set. You can get yours at www.youngliving.com and check with the friend who gave you this book to get the best discount. The following is a list of essential oils used in the Raindrop® Technique in the order listed.

- Valor®
- Oregano
- Thyme
- Basil
- Cypress
- Wintergreen
- Marjoram
- Aroma Siez™
- Peppermint

## WHITE ANGELICA™

White Angelica™ is not a part of the Raindrop® Technique kit but it is considered a valuable part of the process. Many find that it has a wonderful ability to protect the person giving the Raindrop® session from any bad emotions and energy the receiver may have. If you find yourself to be very empathetic with others, this oil is a must. Simply rub one drop over your heart and breathe in deeply prior to inviting the receiver into the room. Then offer some to the receiver as well to protect them in the same way. Rub some on their shoulders at the beginning of the session and allow them to breathe it in before you get started.

## THE BASE

Because this application calls for a lot of essential oils, many of which are considered hot, it is important to start with a base of carrier oil along the back if the receiver is new to the Raindrop® Technique or has more sensitive skin. If you notice any redness on their back and especially their neck, add more carrier oil. V-6™ carrier comes in the kit and is an excellent choice!

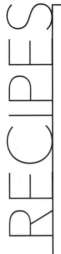

**RECIPES**

### FLUSH WITH H2O

Please don't miss this one. Both the giver and receiver must drink tons of water. If you don't you will end up with a splitting headache. The detox and flushing from this session is very intense. Make sure you drink a minimum of 32 ounces of water within the first hour and continue drinking 16-32 more ounces within the next 2-4 hours or so. Flushing your system with water will help your body benefit from this session without all the harsh detox effects.

### WATER RECIPE

32 ounces infused with 3 drops Lemon Vitality™ and 1 drop Peppermint Vitality™ to help flush your system.

Drink a total of 64 ounces in 4-6 hours to fully flush your system.

# THE BLESSING OF RAINDROP

## LESSON #14

# *LAYERING TECHNIQUE*

Layering is amazing! In the previous lesson we covered the Raindrop Technique®. Did you know that the Raindrop Technique® is a layering technique? Layering is something most people don't know about or don't do. We have gotten used to the fast and easy use of rollerballs. While roll-ons (rollerballs) are great, using a layering method can be incredibly beneficial in a different way. With roll-ons you get a specific synergy that is created...it is something "other" than the sum of its parts. When you layer, you get the benefits of the individual oils (the multiple constituents) one at a time in a specific succession that will blow you away! This lesson will help you get started on your new-found layering journey!

# *HOW TO LAYER*

Layering is a way to place single species oils on your body, one at a time, in a specific order. You can apply them neat or with a carrier depending on the location. If you are layering on the bottom of your feet, you can apply them neat. If you are layering them on your back, you would want to apply a carrier first and also right at the end.

**The Basic instructions:**
1. Add each oil one at a time
2. Rub each oil in for 30-60 seconds before applying the next
3. Use a carrier at the beginning and end for hot oils or just at the end to cap off all the oils to help drive them in.
4. Give yourself a 1-2 minute massage after applying all the oils.

The EO Bar app contains an entire section on Layering. You can find several great recipes to help you on your journey! The EO Bar is available at The App Store and Google Play. For book lovers out there, "French Aromatherapy" contains an entire chapter dedicated to layering! You can get this book on Amazon or buy in bulk over at www.31oils.com/french for your friends and team.

# LAYERING WITH SINGLES

The best way to layer is to choose 3 to 5 essential oil singles that match a profile, yet balance each other. Use a combination of essential oils such as 3 calming oils or 3 strengthening oils and then add a couple more to balance them out. For example, for a healthy immunity, you could layer 3 oils that have a strong affinity toward immunity support with 1 calming oil and 1 flushing oil. So, you might choose Oregano, Clove, and Tea Tree, then add Lavender, and Lemon.

# LAYERING WITH BLENDS

You may have noticed in the Layering Recipes section some recipes called for a blend. Yes, you can layer using blends, but it is recommended that you do not use more than 20% blends in a recipe. If you are using 5 oils, make sure no more than 1 is a blend. If you are layering with 10 oils, make sure no more than 2 are blends. Get it? Layering works best with single species, but sometimes using a very specific synergy is amazing too. Some blends to consider as your first oil placement could be:

- Valor®
- Thieves®
- RC™
- Stress Away™
- PanAway™

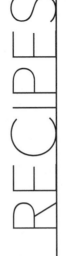

RECIPES

LAYERING

BETTER FOCUS
Application on Back of Neck
1. Copaiba
2. Frankincense
3. Lavender

CALMING
Application on Back of Neck or Wrists
1. Lavender
2. Sacred Frankincense™
3. Vetiver

HEALTH #1
Application on Feet & Back of Neck
1. Frankincense
2. Lavender
3. Oregano
4. Clove
5. Lemon
Note: Use carrier

HEALTH #2
Application on Feet & Back of Neck
1. Thieves®
2. Oregano
3. Tea Tree
4. Frankincense
5. Bergamot
Note: Use carrier

AFTER WORKOUT
Application on Desired Location
1. PanAway®
2. Copaiba
3. Lavender
4. Peppermint
Note: Use carrier

## LESSON #15
# *MAKING ROLL-ONS*

While Layering is amazing, sometimes we just need something super simple and ready-to-go. Enter...the Roll-On. Young Living has created some really incredible Roll-Ons complete with metal fitments. You can get the all-time-favorite Stress Away™ blend in a Roll-On, the seriously necessary Deep-Relief™ Roll-On, the incredibly calming Tranquil™ Roll-On, the night time must, RutaVala™ Roll-On, the perfect Breathe Again™ Roll-On, and don't forget to grab one or 100 of the Valor® Roll-On. These all come ready to use and are pre-diluted with carrier oil. I encourage you to try them all! Another great way to create "grab-and-go" roll ons is to simply add an AromaGlide™ rollerball fitment on any of your favorite essential oil singles or blends. You now have over 200 oil singles and blends to try, let's create some of our own!

# *BLENDS VS SYNERGIES*

Blends are different than synergies, however all synergies are blends. A blend is something that when mixed together you will get the individual therapeutic effects of the oils you have blended. It is like placing 3 different oils into your cold water diffuser one at a time. Every once in a while you might smell one oil, then another, and sometimes a mix of them all. When you create a synergy, you are creating something "other" than the sum of its parts. It is something magical. Take the synergy Thieves® for instance. Every essential oil company on the planet has tried to copy this magical blend and have failed. They don't even come close to the depth and breadth of the action of this oil. They try, but sadly fall short. It is flattering really, but nothing compares to the genuine article! The magic is in the synergy!

A lot goes into making a synergy. Gary Young was an artist at creating them. He was a brilliant "master chef" in the labs of Young Living. For us, it can be a little like "Harry Potter" or the "Mad Scientist" and it makes my heart sing every time I think about how fun it is to play with my oils. The only hard part is when you make something and it sort of isn't great, or is downright bad. That's no fun, because I feel like I have just wasted a bunch of precious oils. So, my goal in this lesson is to help you learn the basics of mixing so you can lessen the mistakes you make.

# MAKING SYNERGIES

I encourage you to play and have fun! The following is a general guideline to follow but is not considered law. You are more than welcome to break these rules, but know, you will generally have more success if you follow them.

1. It is best to work with single species only when you are just starting out.

2. If you want to use a blend, only use one and add 2 or 4 additional singles.

3. It is known that working with 3, 5, or 7 singles makes the most effective synergies.

4. Choose oils within the same family and add 1 or 2 from a different family. (see family groupings list).

5. Once you select your 3, 5, or 7 oils, place them in order from mildest to strongest in aroma. Add them one at a time to a clean dry rollerbottle. Start with only 1 drop of the strongest, then add 2-3 more of each as you go down the line to the mildest. Add more or less of one if you want more of that specific oil aroma.

6. Once you reach the desired aroma, place the cap on and allow the blend to synergize for 24 hours.

7. After it fully synergizes, add some carrier oil or use this synergy to make smaller rollerballs with more carrier. Dilute based on your preference and needs.

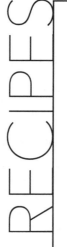

## ROLL-ON RECIPES

Use a 5mL bottle with an AromaGlide™ fitment. Add the oils and allow to synergize for 24 hours then top off with V-6™ oil or the carrier of your choice. These are beginner blends and you may double them if you feel you want or need a stronger dilution ratio. You can see more recipes in the "Rollerball Recipes" section of The EO Bar app.

In drops:

Anger Support
- 10 Bergamot
- 10 Tangerine
- 5 Roman Chamomile

Breathe Support
- 8 Lavender
- 8 Lemon
- 8 Peppermint

Craving Support
- 20 Peppermint
- 10 Lemon

Critter Support
- 10 Tea Tree
- 5 Citronella
- 5 Lemongrass
- 5 Clove
- 5 Melaleuca Quinquenervia

**LESSON #16**

# UNDERSTANDING NOTES

Essential oils tend to group well into categories or families. The following is a general list and many of the oils will cross over into other lists.

## *Top and Middle Notes with Lighter Sweeter Aromas:*

**HIGH IN MONOTERPENES:** Considered stimulating and uplifting. Mostly yellows, oranges, and tans. Lemon, Orange, Tangerine, Grapefruit, Tea Tree, Black Pepper, Frankincense, Fennel, and Cinnamon Bark.

**HIGH IN MONOTERPENE ALCOHOLS and PHENOLS:** Considered stimulating and uplifting. Mostly reds, pinks, and browns. Rose, Bergamot, Geranium, Lavender, Tea Tree, Clove, Oregano, and Thyme.

**HIGH IN ESTERS:** Considered relaxing and soothing. Mostly purples and blues. Roman Chamomile, Clary Sage, Lavender, Wintergreen, and Frankincense.

**HIGH IN ALDEHYDES and KETONES:** Considered cooling and relaxing. Mostly greens. Citronella, Melissa, Lime, Ginger, Lemongrass, Peppermint, Sage, Spearmint, and Thyme, plus others.

## *Middle to Base Notes with Earthier Aromas:*

**HIGH IN SESQUITERPENES:** Considered calming. Mostly blues, purples, and browns. German Chamomile, Clary Sage, Copaiba, Helichrysum, Patchouli, Tansy, and Vetiver.

**HIGH IN SESQUITERPENE ALCOHOLS:** Considered uplifting and calming. Mostly browns. Carrot Seed, Patchouli, Sandalwood, Valerian, and Clary Sage.

# ACTION GROUPS

It can be helpful to group essential oils into "therapeutic action" groupings called action groups. You would place oils that are flushing, such as citrus, in one group, all the oils that are great for health strengthening would be in another group, and all the oils that help with relaxation would be in another group, etc. On the following page is a list that will help you to make your groupings more clear. The oil at the top of each list is the "head of the class" based on the Premium Starter Kit. Once you have your kit, you can add oils to each family grouping so you can start to use your oils more organically. One day you may choose Lemon, and then next day, Orange. One day you may choose Thieves®, and the next day, Clove. To make great roll-ons, try selecting singles from one group to make a powerful synergy or one blend and 2 or 4 singles from the same group.

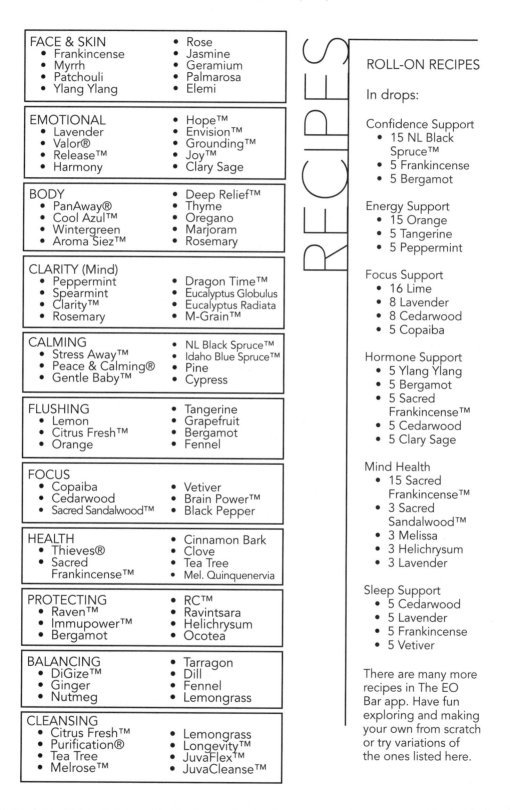

**FACE & SKIN**
- Frankincense
- Myrrh
- Patchouli
- Ylang Ylang
- Rose
- Jasmine
- Geramium
- Palmarosa
- Elemi

**EMOTIONAL**
- Lavender
- Valor®
- Release™
- Harmony
- Hope™
- Envision™
- Grounding™
- Joy™
- Clary Sage

**BODY**
- PanAway®
- Cool Azul™
- Wintergreen
- Aroma Siez™
- Deep Relief™
- Thyme
- Oregano
- Marjoram
- Rosemary

**CLARITY (Mind)**
- Peppermint
- Spearmint
- Clarity™
- Rosemary
- Dragon Time™
- Eucalyptus Globulus
- Eucalyptus Radiata
- M-Grain™

**CALMING**
- Stress Away™
- Peace & Calming®
- Gentle Baby™
- NL Black Spruce™
- Idaho Blue Spruce™
- Pine
- Cypress

**FLUSHING**
- Lemon
- Citrus Fresh™
- Orange
- Tangerine
- Grapefruit
- Bergamot
- Fennel

**FOCUS**
- Copaiba
- Cedarwood
- Sacred Sandalwood™
- Vetiver
- Brain Power™
- Black Pepper

**HEALTH**
- Thieves®
- Sacred Frankincense™
- Cinnamon Bark
- Clove
- Tea Tree
- Mel. Quinquenervia

**PROTECTING**
- Raven™
- Immupower™
- Bergamot
- RC™
- Ravintsara
- Helichrysum
- Ocotea

**BALANCING**
- DiGize™
- Ginger
- Nutmeg
- Tarragon
- Dill
- Fennel
- Lemongrass

**CLEANSING**
- Citrus Fresh™
- Purification®
- Tea Tree
- Melrose™
- Lemongrass
- Longevity™
- JuvaFlex™
- JuvaCleanse™

## RECIPES

## ROLL-ON RECIPES

In drops:

**Confidence Support**
- 15 NL Black Spruce™
- 5 Frankincense
- 5 Bergamot

**Energy Support**
- 15 Orange
- 5 Tangerine
- 5 Peppermint

**Focus Support**
- 16 Lime
- 8 Lavender
- 8 Cedarwood
- 5 Copaiba

**Hormone Support**
- 5 Ylang Ylang
- 5 Bergamot
- 5 Sacred Frankincense™
- 5 Cedarwood
- 5 Clary Sage

**Mind Health**
- 15 Sacred Frankincense™
- 3 Sacred Sandalwood™
- 3 Melissa
- 3 Helichrysum
- 3 Lavender

**Sleep Support**
- 5 Cedarwood
- 5 Lavender
- 5 Frankincense
- 5 Vetiver

There are many more recipes in The EO Bar app. Have fun exploring and making your own from scratch or try variations of the ones listed here.

**LESSON #17**

# ESSENTIAL OILS & PREGNANCY

You may have noticed there is a lot of hype on the internet about safety. Some of it is correct and some of it is incorrect. We have to remember that all products are not created equal. Water is not water when it comes to essential oils. One company's Peppermint may be way too strong or have harmful synthetics in them for women who are pregnant to use, while others are perfectly safe. You will hear people say it is very unsafe to use essential oils neat (without a carrier oil) however that is not true of all oils. Some, like Copaiba, are very mild and are wonderful to use neat on certain areas of the body. A good general rule of thumb of use is: on all walking age humans, all oils may be used neat on the bottoms of the feet. Some areas of the body are more sensitive than others, and some oils are milder or hotter than others. Use common sense and when in doubt go "low and slow." That just means to use them on the bottom of your feet to start and a little at a time with carrier. The fact is, Young Living oils are so pure that most can be used without fear, but always use your noggin!

# DILUTION RATIOS
This is for generally mild oils. For hot oils dilute more.

**Ages 0-1**
1 drop EO to 10 drops carrier, depending on location you may need to dilute more.

**Ages 2-6**
1 drop EO to 4 drops carrier, depending on location you may need to dilute more.

**Ages 7-11**
1 drop EO to 1 drop carrier, depending on location you may need to dilute more.

**Ages 12+**
Use as directed on the label.

# USE WITH CAUTION ON BABIES
- Clary Sage
- Hyssop
- Sage
- Tansy (Tansy is not the same as Blue Tansy. Blue Tansy is perfectly safe)
- Wintergreen
- Eucalyptus Globulus

# ESSENTIAL OIL SAFETY WITH BABIES

Babies have new skin and should always have essential oils applied with carrier oil. In most cases if you are not using a hot oil, you can use a dime size of carrier oil in your palm with one drop of essential oil such as Lavender or Peace & Calming® to rub on their feet and legs. Some moms love applying the mix on the baby's back before bedtime for a calming body massage. There are only a few oils that are to be used with caution with babies, but that does not mean you cannot use them at all. In the case of *Eucalyptus globulus*, it is not that this particular oil is bad, but some people used to practice placing essential oils directly in the nasal cavity to help with stuffiness. This is not recommended for kids or babies because it is too strong of an oil for them in that area. This oil combined into a blend such as RC™ and diffused using 6 drops in a 160mL cold-water diffuser is perfectly safe and actually beneficial. So when you hear to use an oil with "caution" it just means you need to understand the background story.

Many brands can be and are dangerous. The idea that diffusing essential oils around babies is dangerous is based on faulty assumptions. Aromatherapy is the mildest form of essential oil use however, those who claim never to diffuse and never to use essential oils on infants are actually correct in stating that based on the oils THEY use. About 90% of every single oil readily available in the United States is unsafe for infants because they use synthetics or contain fillers that are harmful to babies. Young Living is literally one of the only brands to have zero synthetics in their oils. Did you know that they go far and above any industry standard by doing 20 tests in triplicate two separate times in the process? This is a direct statement from Dr. Buch, Young Living's Chief Science Officer. They do more tests than any other company and each batch is tested using the 20 different tests six times: that is 120 tests on each batch! This is the main reason to never use any brand that does not verify the ENTIRE oil production process from seed selection, to cultivation process, to distillation, to testing, and to bottle sealing.

**LESSON #18**

# *ESSENTIAL OILS & EPILEPSY*

There is a lot of concern around seizures and essential oils. Again, know your company. Most of Young Living's oils have not been noted to cause any issues, however you still need to be your own best advocate.

The following is a list of essential oils to consider avoiding if you are epileptic. These oils contain natural constituents that may be considered neurotoxins that could have a convulsant effect. The convulsant properties are all ketones. It is important to note, that not all ketones are problematic for those with epilepsy. The main ketones to avoid are camphor, thujone, pinocamphone, and fenchone.

- Fenne: 12-16% fenchone containing oil
- Hyssop: 5-17% pinocamphone containing oil
- Rosemary: 6-15% camphor and 1-2% beta-thujone containing oil
- Sage: 4-24% camphor and 18-43% alpha-thujone and 3-8% beta-thujone containing oil
- Spike Lavender (*Lavandula latifolia*): up to 36% camphor containing oil Spike Lavender is not to be confused with Lavender or *Lavandula angustifolia*, which does not contain camphor.
- Tansy (*Tanacetum vulgare*):65-80% beta-thujone and 3-8% camphor containing oil
- Blue Tansy (*Tanacetum annuum*): 10-17% camphor containing oil
- Thuja: thujone containing oil (not a readily available oil)
- Wormwood: thujone containing oil (not a readily available oil)

There is a misconception that any oils containing Eucalyptol are problematic. This comes from the misinterpretation of the oil White Camphor, aka Ravintsara or *Cinnamomum camphora* which does not contain the actual constituent camphor, however its main constituent is 1,8-Cineole which is also called Eucalyptol and is the main constituent in *Eucalyptus globulus*. Therefore, *Eucalyptus globulus* is not problematic for those with epilepsy.

Seizures are triggered by abnormal electrical activity in the brain. Those with epilepsy will not all be affected the same. While this list is a guide it is not to be assumed that you will have a seizure if you use these oils. Furthermore, any synergy or blend that contains a small amount of any of the above oils are even less likely to be problematic. Use your best judgment and consult your physician.

# ESSENTIAL OILS & MEDICATION

There is a long list of essential oils to steer clear of when using prescription medication. This goes back to the issue that most essential oils contain synthetics and fillers. When it comes to using essential oils that are the true, unadulterated botanical, most oils are perfectly safe, save a few as discussed in the next several sections. Please always consult your doctor when considering using essential oils along side of your current medication regimen.

# ESSENTIAL OILS & GRAPEFRUIT JUICE

The Grapefruit Juice Factor is something that people often get hung up on. It is a concern and so I would like to address it. Grapefruit JUICE contains Furanocoumarins which is an inhibitor of enzyme cytochrome P450 3A4 (CYP3A4). This enzyme is an important part of many drugs effectiveness and is necessary to break down the drug. If the drug is inhibited, it will stay in the body longer and potentially cause more side effects.

Essential oils have the ability to stimulate enzyme activity but they do not contain actual enzymes. Grapefruit essential oil contains minor amounts of furanocoumarins (less than 1%). If used as directed, Grapefruit essential oil should not cause any "grapefruit effect" on medications you are using. As with all essential oils, it is important to pay attention to your body and always use based on the bottle label instructions.

Furanocoumarins can be noted by other names as well. Bergapten is a furanocoumarin that is found in expressed Bergamot, but most essential oil companies use furanocoumarin-free Bergamot. You will also find small amounts of bergapten in Neroli (Bitter Orange), Lemon, and Lime essential oils. Bergamottin is a furanocoumarin that is found in Bergamot (again, check to see if your oil is furanocoumarin-free Bergamot), Grapefruit, Lemon and Lime essential oils.

# ESSENTIAL OILS & BLOOD THINNERS

While essential oils will not interact with blood thinners, some will have a similar effect as blood thinners. Each company is different in which oils to stay away from. With Young Living, the oils that may cause increased circulation would be the internal use of Peppermint, Wintergreen, and Oregano. Some oils are pointed out to avoid because of their coumarins which may inhibit the metabolism of medications you are on such as furocoumarin found in Bergamot and Grapefruit essential oils and coumarin in Cinnamon (Cassia, not bark) essential oil. Other times essential oils such as Clove and Nutmeg are singled out due to their excitable nature.

The simple fact is that oils with coumarin or oils that can increase your energy are not a major problem when used as directed. The amount of coumarin found in them is so small that there will be no notable issue felt or seen when using blood thinners. Remember, each person responds differently, so be your own best advocate and pay attention to your body. Diffusing and even the occasional topical application are OK to use while on blood thinners, but please monitor how you feel when using these oils. Every person will respond differently. The most common response with a person on blood thinners who has consumed one drop of Peppermint Vitality™ essential oil, was light-headedness.

# ESSENTIAL OILS & CHEMOTHERAPY

The nature of chemotherapy is that it is a chemical therapy to kill cells. It is a synthetic designed to attack your cells, bad and good. Essential oils are designed to kill chemicals in your body. When you use any essential oil internally they will attack the chemotherapy drug. Most doctors will allow you to use a cold-water diffuser during treatment to help with nausea, but you should not use any oils internally or topically near the cancer area during treatment and up to 24-48 hours after treatment unless your doctor says you can.

# ESSENTIAL OILS & BLOOD PRESSURE

Essential oils don't lower or raise blood pressure in any major way. They can help to dilate arteries, but usually in such small amounts that you won't notice it on your doctor's charts. Essential oils help to balance and support our bodies. If you are not making the right choices in nutrition and exercise, oils will not be able to do their job to their fullest. Consider a house fire. If someone is feeding the fire gasoline on one end and you are trying to put it out on the other end with a garden hose, who do you think will be more successful, the gasoline or the garden hose? It is the same with essential oils. Stop pouring gasoline on your fire so that the garden hose can help.

One of the best ways to help your high blood pressure is to lower your emotional stress. Try any of the calming oils such as Lavender, Frankincense, Sacred Frankincense™, Copaiba, Sacred Sandalwood™, Northern Lights Black Spruce™, Idaho Blue Spruce™, Stress Away™, Peace & Calming®, Valor®, Ylang Ylang, Lime, Tangerine, Clary Sage, Melissa, or Cedarwood.

Contrary to popular belief based solely off of Dr. Jean Valnet's 1964 book, "Aromathérapie", Rosemary, Hyssop, Sage, and Thyme essential oils are safe for people with high blood pressure. Valnet cited several sources that were not conclusive in proving his statement that these four oils cause high blood pressure. Over the past four decades there have been no instances of raised blood pressure of anyone using these oils topically or aromatically. In the study of dogs with internal use of Hyssop through an IV, it was found that in very high doses, enough to cause a seizure in the dog, blood pressure rose just before the seizure then lowered to normal after the seizure.

If you have hypertension, rest assured, essential oils don't raise blood pressure in any major way. Some oils have a safety warning because they have been presumed to raise blood pressure. Essential oils work to balance body systems when used according to instructions.

Always keep in mind, everyone is different, and what works for someone else may not work for you and vice versa. Pay attention to how your body responds. You are your own best advocate!

**LESSON #19**

## *OIL MAPPING*

I coined the term "Oil Mapping" in 2015 because it was the best way to describe what I was doing for my members. In a nutshell, they would tell me all the areas in their life that they wanted to see supported or improved and I would give them tips on how to enhance their routine using essential oils and other lifestyle modifications. As a professional teacher for almost 20 years, I realized early in my career, as do many teachers, that the best way to truly learn something is to teach it. When I decided to start sharing oils with others, I felt it was my duty to understand as much as I could in order to help them. So, I oil mapped! They would give me a list and I would hit the books and research all I could so I could help direct them in the best path. This lesson will help you understand the basics of Oil Mapping and how it can be a win-win for all involved!

You may have little knowledge about essential oils and want to learn more, or you are a seasoned essential oil user who just loves to learn more and more. Either way, Oil Mapping is incredibly fun and rewarding. Oil Mapping considers three main areas in the life of a person: emotional, physical, and mental. Start out by asking the person if they have ever used oils before. Once that is established, ask them if they would like an Oil Map. That always gets lots of questions. Simply share a few common areas where they may be having issues.

Consider using issues that seemingly every person on the planet deals with. Occasionally someone says they are perfect, but usually they say all of the above. Here are the usual three that most people agree they need help supporting: more focus and less stress during the day, better energy to get you through the day, and a more restful nights sleep. Throw in a fun one based on their life stage such as, help with a grumpy husband, or help calming nutty kids. Giving them these examples helps jog their brain. Once they give you a full list, don't be worried about hot words, or medical issues. Your answer will speak above the wellness line.

# HOW TO OIL MAP

Once you have their item list they want support with, get to work doing your research. Make sure you have a really good desk reference and online resources to help you get a larger picture. Be very careful how you answer medical conditions or chronic issues. Since you are most likely not a medical practitioner, it is against the law to give medical advice without a license.

The best way to describe the medical advice issue is to consider the following example: a friend tells you they get headaches all the time and asks for your advice for which oil to use. Perhaps you got a headache last week, and you used Peppermint essential oil on your temples, and it worked great. (Warning: I will go a little dark here, so follow with me.) You tell your friend to do the same. She does and she unexpectedly dies of something not related to the oils. Her husband then searches for why his wife, who died of a brain aneurysm, did not go to the hospital but instead took your advice and used Peppermint. He sues you for deathly advice. He wins.

Even though it was not the oils that caused or even promoted the aneurysm, you are in big trouble because the courts have no way of actually understanding essential oils and the fact that they were not the culprit. While this is a pretty drastic example, I want us all to use common sense and remember this very very important rule of thumb: every human body is different and has underlying issues that stem from multiple system issues, therefore it is not wise to tell someone emphatically what to do for any major health issue.

OK, now that we have that heavy stuff out of the way, my goal is to put a healthy sense of responsibility into your head and heart. We want to help people, not hinder them. The best thing to do is always tell people ahead of time that you will give them ideas to try and here is the key...essential oils help support a healthy body. They do not heal a sick one. When someone tells you they have skin cancer and they ask what oils they should use, it is important that you do not answer what would help with their cancer. You would turn the sick question around and make it a healthy answer such as, "Frankincense and Pine are great oils that help support healthy skin." This is called "above the wellness line" language. Health and wellness, not sickness and disease.

**LESSON #20**

# TERRAIN MAPPING

Terrain Mapping along with the actual implementation of the regimen is one of the hardest yet most rewarding life experiences one can choose to do. The first part is the easy part but knowing is half the battle, right? Let's begin...

# TAKE A LIFE PHOTO

The first part of Terrain Mapping is taking a good long inventory of your life from pre-birth to present. Be super honest with yourself and answer truthfully. The questions below will help get a good "life-photo" of yourself. The goal is to find out what the root cause is for any issues you may be having.

1. What is your family history?

2. Do you have any chronic issues?

3. Any major illnesses or long term medication use?

4. Where were you raised? City or Fresh air?

5. What foods were you fed? Meat and potatoes, lots of milk, processed TV dinners, or fresh ingredients?

6. Were there any power lines or chemicals near your childhood home?

7. What is your current living situation? Healthy area or unhealthy?

8. Are you married? Happily or unhappily?

9. Do you have kids? Do you feel like a good parent or one that needs help?

10. What does your average daily diet look like? Mostly processed or mostly fresh?

11. Do you drink processed beverages of any kind? Soda, tea, flavored drinks? How many?

12. Do you drink coffee? How many cups per day?

13. Do you drink alcohol? How many glasses per day/week?

14. Do you work a stressful job?

15. How many hours per day are you in front of a computer?

16. How many hours per day are you outside?

17. How many minutes per day do you exercise?

18. Do you smoke or take drugs (medicinal or recreational)?

19. How many ounces of straight water do you drink per day?

20. How many servings of fresh fruit do you eat per day?

21. How many servings of fresh veggies do you eat per day?

22. How many grams of animal protein do you eat per day?

23. What supplements are you taking?

24. About how many grams of sugar do you consume each day?

25. Do you pray or meditate every day? How long?

26. How many hours per night do you sleep?

27. Do you wake up refreshed or groggy?

28. Are you often tired during the day?

29. Do you have trouble focusing or multi-tasking?

30. How often do you have a bowel movement?
    What shape and texture is it? What color is your urine?

Answer these questions truthfully to determine your foundation before you can support your long-term health goals.

# BIOFEEDBACK

Now that you know what your foundation looks like, read back over the entire list in the positive. Wipe away the past. Your body needs to know what you want in order to heal. Your mind needs information like a road map. Give it a clear picture. God created our bodies with such intricacies that we may never fully understand. We think a computer is complicated? Our bodies are a gazillion times more complicated than a computer. Just because you may not understand biofeedback fully does not mean it is not real. Create a good photo of your history, then wipe it away. Tell your body you are clean. Tell your body specifically in all the areas you have issues that you are healthy. UPGRADE YOUR VERBAL SOFTWARE!

*Read more about Biofeedback in The EO Bar app under the Education tab.*

# MAKING POSITIVE CHANGES

Making changes is the hardest part of Terrain Mapping. Start with something that you can do, then build on it. Sometimes we do best ripping the bandage off in an "all or nothing" style. If that is you, then go for it! CHOOSE LIFE! But if it would be too overwhelming then work on one thing until you have a handle on it, then go to the next thing. This is basically a life swap. You are going to swap an unhealthy habit for a healthy one. Below are some examples of great Young Living swaps.

*UNHEALTHY FOR HEALTHY*
- Swap coffee for NingXia Red® infused with NingXia Nitro®
- Swap toxic cleaning supplies for Thieves® cleaning supplies, in the laundry, kitchen, bathroom, and whole house!
- Swap toxic face care for ART® system
- Swap synthetic vitamins for the Young Living supplement line
- Swap toxic makeup for Savvy Minerals™
- Swap toxic toothpaste for Thieves® Dentarome Plus
- Swap toxic candles for cold-water diffusers
- Swap uber-toxic air fresheners for natural essential oils
- Swap OTC medicines for healthy alternatives
- Swap toxic energy drinks for NingXia Zyng™
- Swap toxic sunscreen, lotions, hair care, and bug repellent all for Young Living's toxin-free line

It is super simple and cost effective with most YL products either matching or beating the drug-store and department store brands. Contact your rep to find out how to do the swap! You will be so happy you did!

I encourage you to take the Healthy Lifestyle Test on page 150 and watch this very important video to help you understand more on how your body and oils work.

Navigating the Hard Subjects
https://www.facebook.com/JenOSullivanAuthor/
videos/959063170911631/

# NO MORE COFFEE

I realize most people have come up with several reasons why coffee is good for us, but think about that one. Coffee is drastically dehydrating and gives us a false sense of energy. If you are not addicted to the caffeine you are probably addicted to the routine. Coffee has been studied to completely ruin your immune system and lowers your frequency by so much that it puts you in a state of happily accepting all applications for the cold and flu to take residence in your body. No thank you! The following is from the book "French Aromatherapy" and can help you eliminate coffee for good in your life. Coffee addiction is one of the most common struggles that many adults face. To detox from the caffeine in coffee, I recommend the following regimen that will only take about 2 weeks. It's well worth the effort, so I encourage you to try cutting all sources of caffeine out of your life.

1. Take a capsule containing a combination of Peppermint Vitality™ and Dill Vitality™ oils that may help curb your cravings. Blend equal parts in a 5ml bottle then drip 3 drops in an empty capsule and top off with a carrier oil. Take 1–2 of these capsules per day.

2. Drink a gallon of water with 6–12 drops of Lemon Vitality™ essential oil per day. For each 20-24 ounce bottle of water, use 1-2 drops of Lemon Vitality™ essential oil. Add a drop of Peppermint Vitality™ for added craving support.

3. In place of coffee have a warm cup of herbal tea or hot water with fresh lemon and a bit of honey. Try to replace your ritual with something more healthful for your body, such as a cup of hot water with a drop of Thieves Vitality™ and Lemon Vitality™. You can also try "Organic Dandy Blend Instant Herbal Beverage with Dandelion". This is a really healthful alternative!

4. Get your lymphatic system moving by walking for a minimum of 30 minutes a day. If you are up for it, I suggest sweating it out through 60 minutes of rigorous cardio. Also try setting your alarm every hour to remind you to move.

5. Use NingXia Red® and NingXia Nitro® to help replenish and energize your cells.

6. Get a deep tissue massage once a week during detox. After the massage take a hot water bath with 4 cups of Epsom salt. Soak for 20 minutes.

7. Take an Epsom salt bath 3 times a week for 2 weeks. Pour 2–4 cups of Epsom salt into a hot bath and soak your entire body for 20 minutes, which will help regulate the minerals in your body and pull toxins out. Use Dead Sea salt as well. If you use both, do 2 cups of each per bath. Spruce it up with a few drops of Cedarwood and Lavender essential oils.

8. When you feel a craving for coffee, practice deep breathing. Lie down on your back, place your hands on your belly, and take a deep breath to a count of 10 so your lungs fully inflate and your tummy rises. Then breathe out slowly to a count of 20, exhaling as deeply as you can. Try to squeeze all the oxygen out of your lungs. Do this 3–5 times. Get up slowly once you're done.

## LESSON #21
# UNDERSTANDING COMPLIANCE

You may have heard someone say "That's not compliant" or "Sorry, I cannot help you because it would be non-compliant." While some of you know what I am talking about, many of you are saying, "What on Earth is she talking about?" When it comes to the Food and Drug Administration in the United States of America, there are strict guidelines and laws about what companies and those who represent companies can and cannot say. It is not a freedom of speech issue, but rather, it is a safety and false advertising issue. If you do not know if you need to worry about compliance or not ask yourself this question: Do you represent a company that sells products such as makeup, lotion, essential oils, pharmaceuticals, supplements, or food items?

If your answer is yes, then you must follow the FDA rules and guidelines in how you represent the products your company carries. If you are just a customer and do not sell the products yourself, then you are allowed to speak freely, but I would still caution you for your own liability protection. It is important to have an understanding of FDA compliance, even if the subject matter is a bit heavy. I hope I don't bore you, but really, I love this stuff! Why? Because it makes me a much better researcher and advocate for the products I represent!

Things you CAN say: https://www.youtube.com/watch?v=9GLGJVkEj1g&feature=youtu.be

Things you CAN'T say: https://www.youtube.com/watch?v=XTxUOEH4amE&feature=youtu.be

If you are someone who does not sell essential oils or any products governed by the FDA, I still would like you to consider your own personal liability. Friends giving friends advice is very common practice. You would not be a friend if you did not share help. But we all know we need to be smart when we share. Whenever I give advice to a friend and it doesn't work out for them I feel horrible. That does not mean I should stop giving advice. It just means I need to make sure my advice is sound, well thought-out, and wise. Sharing who cuts my grass is different than sharing how to help a medical condition.

Why can doctors make such wild claims sometimes with what seems to be a rabbit hole of an exploration of various treatments and in the end it seems like you are no better off than when you started, or are worse off? They pay thousands upon thousands of dollars on what is called Professional Liability Insurance. If you get hurt while they are "practicing" medicine on you, and you sue them, they are covered. If you give advice to a friend and it goes awry and they sue you, then you will be the one up the river without the proverbial paddle. So be clear and be wise.

## WHAT EXACTLY IS COMPLIANCE?

The FDA has regulated what distributors of an essential oil company can and cannot say to their customers. The term used for this is "compliance". This is for your protection as a distributor. It may feel like you are being handcuffed, but it is important to understand the blessing that working compliantly within your business brings. Compliance may be a new concept for you since we live in a world where freedom of speech matters. Consider this simple transaction between you and a friend who has not used essential oils before. Your friend has a raging migraine. She asks if you have any oil that may help. You personally have found Peppermint to work well for you, so you gladly give her some to try. A couple hours later your friend tells you it didn't work. Just as she suspected– oils don't work and she then decides oils are a sham. The issue here is, you do not know why she has a migraine. It could be from hormones, or dehydration, or perhaps the 9 cups of coffee she has consumed that day. The point is, oils do not work the same way as pharmaceuticals do. Essential oils work organically in our bodies to help support health, not cure illness. A more serious claim could land you in a lawsuit where the court will rule against you simply because there is not enough information on essential oils. The reality is, if you operate your business and disregard compliance, your account will get shut down by Young Living. It is to protect the company as a whole. If one of their distributors is overtly non-compliant, the FDA could step in and shut down the company. Young Living will give you a warning and will work with you to help you clean up anything you are doing incorrectly. They want you to succeed, but it is best to start off on the right foot to begin with.

# HOW TO LEARN IN A WORLD OF COMPLIANCE

This all begs the question, "How can I find out good information on the products even if it is non-compliant?" This is a great question and is actually easily answered! As a distributor, we are not allowed to say something will treat or prevent or even cure something, but we all have had amazing experiences and testimonials about using our products. Not everyone is a representative of the company and so there is a ton of information available right at your fingertips! Here are just a few resources for those of you who really want to understand what proven properties and actions essential oils contain! There are apps and books you can purchase. Ask your enroller what books they recommend that are from verified third parties that will give you the CORRECT information. Beware of info that is incorrect based on our way of using oils and Young Living's oils. They are different and are used differently.

I also encourage you to take a class if you are REALLY getting into it all. Not just any class, but a class through a certified school on the subject of essential oils. I have researched many schools and the one that I have found to be far and above the best is The New York Institute of Aromatic Studies. While getting a formal education is not necessary, it sure is fun. Good thing they also offer free courses as well as low investment more in-depth courses. The ones I recommend are:

French Foundations
This is a Level One Aromatherapy Certification and is a prerequisite for getting your Full Aromatherapy Certification. It is all online and works as a go at your own pace schedule. It takes around 3-6 months to complete. You can find more information and group discounts at www.Facebook.com/groups/TheHumanBody

Other resources include reference guides of which there are many and online testimonial searches. I caution you to be your own best health advocate and remember what worked for one person may not work for you!

# HOW TO SHARE COMPLIANTLY

Here are some tips to keep both you and your customers happy.

- Talk about oils from a health perspective. This is called speaking "above the wellness line"and is a great way to shift your focus.

- Never use any words that imply or claim sickness. Examples: cold, flu, sick, cough, sore throat, infection, virus, bacteria, inflammation, pain, under-the-weather, headache, head-in-a-vice, heartburn, high blood pressure, constipation, etc. See the "hot words" list in Appendix B on page 152.

- Never use any words that are clearly diseases or names for disorders. Examples: Cancer, Eczema, ADD/ADHD, or any autoimmune disorder such as MS, Lyme, FM, RA, etc. See the "hot words" list in Appendix B on page 152.

- FDA Guidelines state that a product may not be labeled for topical and aromatic use as well as for consumption. Structure function claims, such as respiratory, digestive, circulatory claims, are only permissible for dietary supplements. When making system function claims, only refer to the Vitality™ line of consumable essential oils in the United States.

- Never share links to other websites on your own website or on any social media platforms. Example: do not share a recipe from another website and link that website. It is better to copy and paste the recipe and give credit to the website name without the dot com at the end. The reason for this is if the website you link to has any non-compliant information on it at all, you are also liable.

- Do not give out non-compliant information to your customers at the time of sale. You may direct them to third party resources (see The Resources page) to help them in their own research or suggest they take a free course at The New York Institute of Aromatic Studies.

- Always remind your customers that essential oils help support health, not cure, treat, or heal sickness and disease.

# UPGRADE YOUR VERBAL SOFTWARE

Many years ago I had my friend Simon T. Bailey speak at one of my master-mind coaching group sessions. As usual he blew me away. I remember one clever phrase he used that has stuck with me all these years. "Upgrade your verbal software!" We are constantly having to upgrade apps and computer software, but when it comes to our own lives I feel like we often forget to upgrade. We are more on a path of a slow downgrade with viruses and bugs getting in until we wake up one morning only to realize we are out of commission and our system has completely crashed.

I'm a complainer, or better phrased, I'm a "recovering complainer". We should create a group of Complainers Anonymous but I fear we'd just spur one another on toward hate and bad deeds. As a recovering complainer I try to steer clear of others who complain like the plague! No thank you! I'm not interested in that drama anymore! What's interesting about upgrading your verbal software is when you start paying attention to your words... like REALLY pay attention... Stop. No. Bad. Sorry. Debt. Sick. Tired. Overwhelmed. Can't. Don't. Busy. Freaked out. Crazy. Uggg... you'll notice all of these words are negative.

How often do you say you're too busy? Or overwhelmed? Or how about the word "sorry"? Change it up! Stop saying it in the negative. See there, I said stop. That's negative. I should say, "Consider saying it in the positive" rather than "Stop saying it in the negative." It's a simple shift but can make a radical difference in your life! Here are a few examples.

"My goal this year is to become debt free!"
*A better way of saying this would be:*
**"My goal this year is to become financially free!"**

"I'm sick and tired of being sick and tired!"
*A better way of saying this would be:*
**"Today I choose to be healthy!"**

"I'm so sorry for being late!"
*A better way of saying this would be:*
**"Thank you for being patient."**

"I'm so busy!"
*A better way of saying this would be:*
**"I've been very productive lately!"**

"Life has been overwhelming lately!"
*A better way of saying this would be:*
**"God has given me a great season of growth."**

When you continually speak in the negative, you continually bring about negative energy and negativity will follow you wherever you go. Have you ever noticed your friends who are in constant turmoil? They are the ones constantly complaining! The opposite is true for those who have a positive outlook on life and who are using positive words filled with cheer and gratitude. Things always seem to go right for them! Hmmm...very interesting!

Something even more interesting has happened in the past several years with the regulatory compliance shift when the FDA stepped in and asked us all as essential oil distributors to speak compliantly. For those of you new to the term "compliance" it means a distributor of essential oils is unable to make health claims such as an oil will cure, treat, or heal any disease or illness. Giving a simple diagnosis and treatment idea to a friend who has a headache and then recommending an oil to help, would be considered medical advice and you could be sued for "practicing medicine without a license". It's serious stuff!

Guess what compliance is? It's an upgrade in our verbal software. Instead of talking about disease and illness, compliance has forced us to upgrade our verbal software and talk about health and wellness. Some of you have decided to side-step compliance and talk disease and sickness behind closed doors. I encourage you to consider compliance an upgrade. Otherwise you're continuing the negative cycle. When I talk about fruits and veggies to help keep me healthy it's the same thing. I talk about oils to keep me healthy. It's part of my lifestyle change. Fruits. Veggies. Essential oils. Exercise. More water. Less of all the bad stuff. Get it?

*Bad for you stuff:* Processed foods, medications, processed white sugar, alcohol, drugs, tobacco, coffee (basically anything that will cause addiction), negative people.

*Good for you stuff:* Fruits, veggies, whole foods, essential oils, exercise, water, sunshine (being in clean air), happy people.

So who's ready to shift their life in a more positive healthy direction! Who's ready to choose Vitality! Let's start a Vitality lifestyle revolution!! Are you in? #ChooseVitality

# LESSON #22
# THE MAGIC OF THIEVES®

Thieves®: that wonder of all wonders! Have you tried it yet? No, not the oil! The full line of products?! It will blow anything you are currently using out of the water! One little capful lasts sooooo long and cleans everything. Say goodbye to a bin full of random cleaning solutions and hello to one neat and tidy bottle of Thieves® Household Cleaner. Ditch all those toxins in your personal care items and swap them out with the Thieves® toothpastes, mouth wash, floss, hand soap, bar soap, waterless hand purifier, laundry detergent, automatic dishwasher powder, dish soap, fruit & veggie soak and spray, wipes, portable spray, and don't forget the cough drops, hard lozenges, and mints! Do the ditch & switch! Literally ditch all your toxins in one fell swoop and switch everything out to the Thieves® line!

The Thieves® line is worth sharing with everyone! Did you know you can sign up to be a wholesale member by getting only the Thieves® Premium Starter Kit? Ask your enroller about how to share. If you know someone who is obsessed with cleaning and you think they could benefit from this beautifully clean line of products, then start sharing it with them. Who knows, it could make all the difference in their healthy life!

# FUN WITH THIEVES®

The name "Thieves" comes from a legend about four thieves who rubbed on a similar blend before they robbed the dead and dying during the plague. This blend contains 5 single oils: Clove, Lemon, Cinnamon Bark, Eucalyptus Radiata, and Rosemary.

This synergy is amazingly good at cleaning pretty much everything and anything! I encourage you to try the whiteboard test. Get a white dry erase board, draw on it with permanent marker, then drip a drop of Thieves® essential oil on it and watch the magic! It is truly a wonder! Let's see how we can incorporate it into our lives.

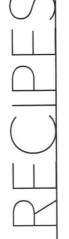

## *GET ALL THE THIEVES®*

Don't start small...just wipe out every toxin in your home once and for all. Toss it all! Guess what? It will only be an investment of around $400 but you will get a whopping $800 worth of items! Head over to your membership account online and sign up for Essential Rewards just for this month. I will share with you about Essential Rewards in the next class, but trust me, this will be worth it and you can cancel at anytime. Add the following to your ER order and you will get all the amazing free promos this month! Such an incredible deal!

Premium Starter Kit with Thieves®
- Thieves® Dish Soap
- Thieves® Laundry Soap
- Thieves® Automatic Dishwasher Powder
- Thieves® Dentarome Ultra Toothpaste
- Thieves® AromaBright Toothpaste
- Thieves® Dental Floss
- Thieves® Hard Lozenges
- Thieves® Cough Drops
- Thieves® Foaming Hand Soap 3 Pack
- Thieves® Mints
- Thieves® Wipes
- Thieves® Fruit & Veggie Spray

### DIFFUSER

Some people absolutely LOVE Stress Away™ but want to try it without the Vanilla absolute. Here is a very simple version of this beloved oil that you can try in your cold-water diffuser.

- 2 drops Copaiba
- 3 drops Lavender
- 3 drops Cedarwood
- 6 drops Lime

### TOPICAL

Sacred Sandalwood™ rubbed on the front of the throat is a divine experience. Try it and you will quickly find out why! The sesquiterpenes are heavier and allow this beautiful oil to stay with you all day long!

# DITCH & SWITCH

## LESSON #23
# *TRULY TOXIC-FREE MAKEUP*

I am so thrilled to finally find a toxic-free makeup line. So many companies claim they are "clean" but use talc, a known carcinogen, or bismuth, a highly reactive ingredient to many who have sensitive skin. I was skeptical at first since I do have very sensitive skin and I want to set it and forget it. Savvy Minerals has been fundamentally incredible and surprisingly effective! This lesson is dedicated to some fun tips and tricks when it comes to using Savvy Minerals! The following are the chemical count found in many toxic cosmetics:

- 168 chemicals in makeup
- 26 chemicals in eyeshadow
- 16 chemicals in blush
- 33 chemicals in lipstick

Are you ready to make the Savvy Switch? The FDA has stated, "Our data show that over 99% of the cosmetic lip products and externally applied cosmetics on the U.S. market contain lead at levels below 10 ppm." While 10 ppm may seem low, the issue is that we reapply and reapply plus the addition of other personal care products that contain trace amounts until finally we realize we are poisoned by lead and don't even know it. Let's just choose to use lead-free lipstick!

## *PURITY & COSMETICS*

Young Living was founded on an important principle: never skimp on purity. This principle is deeply ingrained into every product Young Living creates. Savvy Minerals™ is a truly magical product that is both gorgeous on and healthy for your skin. To get great tips, please join our tutorial group at www.SavvyFace.com (www.Facebook.com/groups/savvyface) or head over to www.SavvyMinerals.com for the full story behind the makeup!

## *MAKEUP TIPS*

### *LIP TIPS*
All lip colors work well together. Consider if you wear more plums, pinks, or beiges and select accordingly. Pro Tip: For lip liner, try Passionate blush using a little water and a lining brush. For darker color play with mixing the Multitasker with shimmer eyeshadow, apply wet, then add gloss.

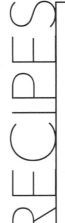

### FOUNDATION TIPS

The Cool and Warm tones are for paler toned women. Check the veins on your wrists in natural daylight. If blue, and you burn easily, then you are in the Cool family. If green, and you tan easily, you are in the Warm family. If you find you are somewhere in the middle go with Warm. Cool are pink tones, Warm are yellow tones. The Dark set is for darker toned women and all have a warm tone to them. Pro tip: For fuller coverage, spritz your brush with Misting Spray and dip into foundation, then apply to face. For more sheer coverage, use the foundation dry using small circular motions to blend in well. All makeup is buildable to your desired look. For the color selection chart and more tips on how to use the Foundation, go to www.SavvyMinerals.com

### BLUSH TIPS

If you are lighter in tone, use one of the pink or plum shades. If you are darker in tone, consider using the darker plum shade, a bronzer, or a darker shade of foundation.

### EYESHADOW TIPS

Choose from mattes or shimmers or a blend of both. The Multitasker is a must for eyeliner, shadow, brow-liner, and gray hair coverage. For basics, choose a highlight, a pink/plum medium, and a darker contouring shadow. Use foundation wet as a concealer. Don't forget the eyeliner!

**89**

### PRODUCT HACKS

Hacks make life interesting and useful. Here are a few to try:

- MultiTasker to darken your lipstick
- MultiTasker to color gray hair
- Darker Blush as lip liner
- Dark Foundations for contouring
- Dark Foundations as bronzer
- Blushes as eyeshadow
- Seedlings Wipes to clean brushes
- Thieves® Household Cleaner to deep clean brushes
- LavaDerm™ Cooling Mist if Misting Spray is out of stock
- Best Kept Secret with ART® Light Moisturizer as concealer
- Wanderlust or Veil to build long full lashes
- Lavender Lip Balm as eyelid primer

For more on how to do these hacks go to www.SavvyFace.com

## LESSON #24
# *FACE SUPPORT*

One thing people love when they first buy a kit, is how they learn to change their face regimen. Honestly, it is so simple, yet so amazing, that they all wonder why on Earth they never knew about this before! This lesson will cover everything to do for a flawless face BEFORE you apply your makeup. The Savvy Minerals line is amazeballs for glamming it up, but having a great canvas is equally important. Let's redefine our face regimen!

# *GREAT SKIN*

Great skin starts from the inside out. Too many of us have opted to drink reverse osmosis water or fully filtered bottle water and have depleted our body of vital minerals. Young Living states, "Mineral Essence™ is a balanced, full-spectrum ionic mineral complex enhanced with essential oils. According to two-time Nobel Prize winner Linus Pauling PhD., 'You can trace every sickness, every disease, and every ailment to a mineral deficiency.' Ionic minerals are the most fully and quickly absorbed form of minerals available."

Your skin thrives in a more alkaline environment. The more fruits and veggies you consume, the more antioxidants you place into your system to help battle those pesky free-radicals. You'll want to choose more color, too! If you can get a good rainbow color variety in your meal, you are much better off. Forget the bland plate of white meat, white potatoes, yellow corn, and pale pasty iceberg lettuce. Go with bold, bright, and beautiful colors. Your skin loves dark leafy greens, too!

If you really want to help alkalize your body, take AlkaLime™ every day. Young Living states, "AlkaLime® is a precisely-balanced alkaline mineral complex formulated to neutralize acidity and maintain desirable pH levels in the body. Infused with Lemon and Lime essential oils and organic whole lemon powder, AlkaLime also features enhanced effervescence and biochemic cell salts for increased effectiveness. A balanced pH is thought to play an important role in maintaining overall health and vigor."

## DETOX WITH WATER

It is very important that you consider upping your water game and adding back in some nutrients. Water is the key to helping rid your body of free-radicals. These free-radicals cause oxidative stress on your body and most noticeably your skin. The average person needs to drink 50% of their bodyweight in ounces each day. If you are wanting to flush your body, you will want to reach for 60-75% of your bodyweight in ounces.

Water per day:

- If you are 100-125lbs try to drink around 60-90 ounces per day.

- If you are 125-150lbs try to drink around 90-115 ounces per day.

- If you are 150-200lbs try to drink around 100-125 ounces per day.

- If you are over 200lbs, please consult your doctor. Drinking a gallon a day will help you shed some pounds.

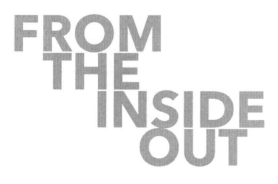

FROM THE INSIDE OUT

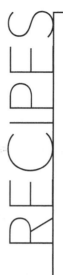

RECIPES

DELUXE EYE SERUM

One of my most beloved recipes is called "No Crow" because it helps us to not have those crazy crow's feet! You will love this one...and, no, you cannot sub anything from this recipe. If you have to beg or borrow some of these to make this, it will be well worth it.

- 15 drops Gentle Baby™
- 15 drops Sacred Frankincense™
- 15 drops Myrrh
- 9 drops Patchouli
- 3 drops Rose

Add all essential oils to a 15 mL glass dropper bottle, swirl to blend, then add 1/4 bottle Rosehip Seed oil, and 3/4 bottle Jamaican Black Castor oil.

# FACE CLEANSING ROUTINE

Yep, I get it. You need to have a squeaky clean face. But seriously, who ever told you that is what you need to have? Did you ever stop to think that you are stripping your skin of its own natural healing and regenerating properties? I am going to offer up an alternative to a soapy, squeaky clean face. Just use water. Say what? Come again? Did you just say, ONLY WATER? Why, yes I did.

I want you to go buy a really good quality microfiber face cloth. You can get them from any beauty store. Any microfiber cloth will do, but it is best to find one that is higher quality. Get it nice and warm and wet, place it over your dirty face at the end of the day, and wipe clean. Here is the issue: cleaning with a microfiber cloth takes more time and patience. It will remove all of your makeup but you need to let the microfiber do its thing.

Here is how you use it: Get it wet with warm to slightly hot water, place the cloth directly onto your closed eye, let sit for 30 seconds, then wipe off makeup. Keep wiping gently until all makeup is removed. Using a microfiber cloth takes more time because you need to clean your face (wipe it fully down) 3-4 times, but your skin will love you for it. Bye bye soap! Hello gorgeous glowing skin!

OK, OK, so I realize sometimes you need a deep clean. For that I recommend the ART® Gentle Cleanser from Young Living. This foaming cleanser is gentle enough for those of you who can't bear the thought of NOT using a cleanser and is amazing for your skin!

# FACE CARRIER OILS

Using straight up carrier oil, as in greasy, oily oil, helps balance out your skin! Carrier oils such as V-6™, grapeseed, sweet almond, and rosehip seed oil are known for their skin beautifying properties. Even Cleopatra was known to lather her whole body in almond oil. This is not something new, but science has got our heads all tangled up in the "beauty is better through science" approach. Didn't our mothers always say, "simple is always better"? Consider creating your own concoction to use with your skin type for the perfect face serum. Once you try it, you will never go back!

# FACE SUPPLEMENTS

You most likely need to get more minerals, more water, and more fruits and veggies. So start with that great foundation. But I also know, many of you have a hard time drinking that much water and getting that many fruits and veggies mixed into your daily routine. Here are a few tips to help you out.

- Use NingXia Red® to get a great blend of nutrients for anti-oxidative support. You will want to drink 2-4 ounces per day for the first 4 weeks to detox, then you can step it down to 2 ounces per day.

- Use MultiGreens™ capsules to fill in the veggie gap. Made with spirulina, alfalfa sprouts, barley grass, bee pollen, eleuthero, Pacific kelp, and therapeutic-grade essential oils, MultiGreens™ is a must for every human!

- Add citrus Vitality™ oils to your water. Get a stainless steel or glass water bottle and add 1-4 drops of any of your favorite citrus Vitality™ oils. Mix and match and don't forget to play a bit with 1 drop of Peppermint Vitality™ or Spearmint Vitality™ every so often!

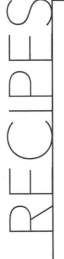

THE KING OF OILS

Frankincense is one of the most versatile oils on the planet. Theory states that it was given to Jesus as a toddler by one of the Three Wise Men as a symbol. Frankincense was often used as an embalming ingredient in ancient Egyptian times. Symbolism was and still is a very large part of Eastern life. It would make sense that the Wise Men would offer this symbol as a gift to the child who came to ultimately die. Frankincense is a great oil to use for calming and meditation, but it is amazing to help preserve our skin.

- Add one drop of Frankincense every day to your normal face cream.

- Dab a bit of Frankincense around aged areas on the face after you apply your cream or serum.

- Use a drop on the back of your hands daily and apply carrier oil on top.

**LESSON #25**

# FACIAL CARE PRODUCTS

Facial care support with ready-made products is often what is called for when you don't have a lot of time. In the previous lesson I covered some DIY products as well as the foundation to great skin. In this lesson, let's be real, 'cuz who has time to make DIY stuff all the time. Yes, mama said simple is best, and Young Living has cornered the market on creating the most amazing products that are so clean and simple and ohhhhh sooooo effective! You are going to love these products because they fill your deep ingrained desire for a multi-step system as well as your new found love for everything toxin free! Yippee!!!

## ART® SKIN CARE SYSTEM

Yes and yes! This is the easiest and best way to get started. Cleanser, Toner, and Moisturizer. Done and done. "Young Living's ART® Skin Care System safely and effectively cleanses, tones, and moisturizes your face to bring out your natural and inherent beauty. That is the beauty of ART®!"

Here's how it works: The cleanser gently lifts the dirt and makeup from your face by opening your pores and allowing the water to wash it from the surface. The toner helps to close the pores back up and tone them to help minimize their appearance. The moisturizer adds the perfect amount of rejuvenating moisture back to your face. This system is perfect for any and all skin types and any and all ages. This is as easy and clean as it gets. Heads up though, if you have been using over-the-counter face products or even the more expensive department store brands, beware, your skin will go through a detox period as these products gently pull out all the damaging toxins over the next month. So be consistent and stay the course. Within just a few weeks your skin will start to feel and look healthier.

### CLEANSE
We know soaps strip our faces of natural oils. Using the Orange Blossom Facial Wash is a great way to wash your face without the harsh soap experience. "This gentle, soap-free facial wash cleanses the skin without stripping natural oils. It contains MSM for softening and Lavender essential oil to soothe skin." ~ Young Living

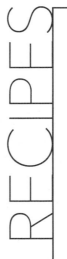

## EXFOLIATE

Everyone needs a good scrub once in a while. Use this scrub once a week to gently scrub away excess skin cells. Satin Facial Scrub is a water-based exfoliant that contains ingredients to minimize the appearance of pores and invigorate dull skin.

## RENEW

Have you tried the ART® Renewal Serum yet? It not only smells amazing but it is so nurturing! "ART® Renewal Serum is an intricate blend of exotic orchid extract and essential oils that benefits the most delicate areas of the face. These premium ingredients are formulated to deeply nourish, hydrate, and help maintain a youthful appearance." ~ Young Living

I encourage you to get this as a primer for your Savvy Minerals. It helps those minerals stay put all day long. Just a little all over your face just before you apply your makeup and you are good to go!

## HYDRATE

Some of us need just a bit more hydration at night. The ART® Intensive Moisturizer is just the ticket! This is truly luxurious and smells so amazing you will want to use it every single day! A little goes a long way so this decadence will last you a while. Once again, another product derived completely from natural ingredients. Say goodbye to toxins! We've declared war!

## REPAIR

Remember having a slumber party and raiding your mom's medicine cabinet for her coveted masque? We'd all sit around with our faces covered in slime laughing at how ridiculous we looked. So much fun! Young Living has created two masques that you are sure to fall in love with! The ART® Beauty Masque that is a full masque you apply to your face and the ART® Creme Masque that you smooth over your face. Both you leave on for 20 minutes for a spa-like finish to your beautiful face!

**THE PERFECT REGIMEN:**

WASH: Morning and night with Orange Blossom Facial Wash or the ART® Gentle Face Wash.

SCRUB: 1-2 times a week with Satin Facial Scrub™.

TONE: Morning and night with the ART® Refreshing Toner.

BRIGHTENER: If needed, Sheerlume™ is to be used first under all other products to help brighten and balance skin tones.

SERUM: Morning and night with the ART® Renewal Serum.

MOISTURIZE: Morning with the ART® Light Moisturizer. Night with the ART® Intensive Moisturizer.

REPAIR: Once a week with the ART® Creme Masque.

**LESSON #26**

# THE ANSWER TO TOXIC BABY PRODUCTS

The Seedlings™ product line is an answer to the often asked question, "What is safe to use on my baby?" As a mom myself, this question is what originally drove me to Young Living in 2007. The Seedlings™ has transformed how we as moms see baby products. I am not interested in formaldehyde in my baby's shampoo. Did you know formaldehyde was a very common preservative used in shampoos? While most companies have cleaned up their act, it can be quite a guessing game when it comes to baby products. With Young Living you can rest assured that every product from the Seedlings™ line contains only ingredients known to be safe for use on infants.

Here is a short list of items commonly found in many baby products that are known carcinogens, endocrine disruptors, and gene mutators:
- Talc
- Parabens
- Mineral Oil
- Propylene Glycol
- 1,4-dioxane Surfactant
- Ethylated Surfactant
- Triclosan
- Synthetic Fragrance

## SEEDLINGS™ BABY WIPES

The products from the Seedlings™ line are not only the perfect choice for babies, but also for adults. The Baby Wipes can be used to remove makeup, to clean makeup brushes, as face refresher cloths, and personal toilet wipes (don't flush down the toilet please). They smell amazing and both you and your baby will love them! Here is what Young Living says about them, "Specially developed for infants' delicate skin, these wipes use pure essential oils for babies and cleansing botanicals in a mild formula with a clean and soothing scent. Made from soft, durable fibers, these gentle baby wipes thoroughly clean from head to toe, while leaving skin smooth and smelling sweet."

## SEEDLINGS™ BABY LOTION

Oh so good for your baby and also makes a great face and body lotion for adults too! Young Living states, "Nourish baby's delicate skin with a lightly scented, plant-based moisturizer that uses pure essential oils for infants in its gentle formula. This mild lotion quickly absorbs into the skin to gently moisturize, smooth, and support healthy-looking skin."

# SEEDLINGS™ BABY WASH & SHAMPOO

If you have sensitive skin, this is the best body wash for people of all ages! The Seedlings™ Baby Wash & Shampoo is an all-in-one, easy to use product for baby and you. Young Living states, "Made specifically for baby's needs, Young Living Seedlings™ Baby Wash & Shampoo gently cleanses skin and hair, leaving it soft, smooth, and lightly scented with Young Living's Calm blend of Lavender, Coriander, Bergamot, Ylang Ylang, and Geranium. Comprised of the purest ingredients and essential oils for babies, the sulfate-free, non-drying formula is also tear-free and ready for bath time play."

# SEEDLINGS™ DIAPER RASH CREAM

So many of Young Living's products may be used for what we call "life hacks". It is where you find a great product and discover another use for it. In the case of the Diaper Rash Cream, you can use it to protect you and your baby's skin when out in the sun for a longer amount of time. The 14% Zinc Oxide is a natural skin protectant. Young Living states, "Young Living's Seedlings™ Diaper Rash Cream gently rubs onto infants' skin to relieve, treat, and prevent diaper rash. Created with the purest naturally derived ingredients for your baby, the formulation of essential oils, soothing botanicals, and non-nano zinc oxide reduces redness, seals out wetness, protects the skin, and provides immediate relief on contact."

# SEEDLINGS™ BABY OIL

Once again, another product for both you and your baby! Use this oil to pamper your freshly shaved legs and also your baby's healthy skin wherever it is needed. Young Living states, "Formulated specifically for infants, Young Living Seedlings™ Baby Oil moisturizes, soothes, and nourishes delicate skin with plant-based ingredients and baby-safe essential oils. Use it throughout the day or as part of a nighttime routine to promote a restful night's sleep with its peaceful, relaxing scent."

# SEEDLINGS™ LINEN SPRAY

Use this spray everywhere and anywhere! It is the safest, fresh-smelling air and fabric freshener you can buy! Young Living states, "Envelop your child in the calming aroma of Young Living Seedlings™ Linen Spray. This naturally derived spray uses infant-safe essential oils but no alcohol, artificial fragrances or dyes, or synthetic preservatives, so it safely freshens bedding, car seats, and clothing throughout everyday play and nighttime routines."

**LESSON #27**

# THE WONDERS OF NINGXIA RED®

The moment you get your Premium Starter Kit, you open it up like a kid on a holiday! Oh the wonders! But wait! There's more!? Under the oils there is a little hidden panel that takes you to a whole new world! NingXia! What are those little red packets? I remember getting my kit and not even knowing what to do with them. I don't think I even tried them for several months!!! Yikes! Looking back, I had no clue what amazingness was to be had with those two little packets. So, go to your kit if you still have them in there, pop them in the fridge, then read up in this lesson on why you NEED those packets and how they may just change your life for the better!

# WHAT IS NINGXIA RED®?

NingXia Red® is a whole body supplement for a more healthful life experience. The wolfberry, also known as the goji berry, is touted for having high antioxidant properties. A daily shot helps support better energy and normal cellular function, as well as whole-body health and wellness. Four ounces of NingXia Red® equals one serving of fruit; however, one ounce has the antioxidant equivalent to eating 4lbs of carrots or 8 whole oranges!

Fun facts about NingXia Red®: The Orange, Yuzu, Lemon, and Tangerine essential oils in NingXia Red® contain d-limonene, which is a powerful wellness-promoting constituent. NingXia Red® is free of high fructose sweeteners. Wolfberries and exotic fruits such as blueberry, cherry, aronia, pomegranate, and plum give NingXia Red® its delicious flavor.

"Young Living NingXia Red® benefits include support for energy levels, normal cellular function, and whole-body and normal eye health. A daily shot of 2–4 ounces helps support overall wellness with powerful antioxidants." ~ Young Living

INGREDIENTS: Proprietary NingXia Red® Blend 29g, NingXia Wolfberry Puree, Blueberry Juice Concentrate, Plum Juice Concentrate, Cherry Juice Concentrate, Aronia Juice Concentrate, Pomegranate Juice Concentrate Proprietary Essential Oil blend 50mg, Grape seed extract, Orange, Yuzu, Lemon, Tangerine. Other ingredients: Tartaric acid, natural blueberry flavor, pure vanilla extract, malic acid, pectin, sodium benzoate/natural stevia extract.

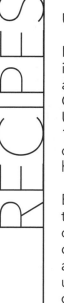

# WOLFBERRIES

Wolfberries are also known as Goji berries "The wolfberries sourced for NingXia Red® hail from the Ningxia province in northern China. This superfruit has one of the highest percentages of fiber of any whole food and contains zeaxanthin—a carotenoid important to maintaining healthy vision. It also contains polysaccharides, amino acids, and symbiotic vitamin mineral pairs that when present together promote optimum internal absorption. By using whole wolfberry puree—juice, peel, seeds, and fruit—Young Living is able to maintain more of the desired health-supporting benefits in every bottle of NingXia Red." - Young Living

## SERVING SIZE

BOTTLES: NingXia Red® Bottles give you just about 25 servings and allows you the flexibility to drink more or less as needed.

2oz PACKETS: NingXia Red® Packets are perfect to throw in your purse or take anywhere on the go. You may drink them at room temperature or chill them (I like them best chilled). One or two packets per day and you are good to go!

## SAFETY

NingXia Red® is safe for all people from solid-food eating children to adults. Pregnant and nursing women should also consider using NingXia Red® as part of their healthy daily regimen.

### USAGE IDEAS

NingXia Red® is a must for all humans! Common Uses: Drink 1-4 ounces daily to support health.

Best Practice: In the morning, drink one ounce of NingXia Red® alone or mix it up and add one drop of Thieves Vitality™ or Frankincense Vitality™. In the afternoon, drink one ounce and add one drop of Tangerine Vitality™ or Longevity Vitality™ or any oil from the Vitality™ line.

# NINGXIA® INFUSED PRODUCTS

NingXia Red® is a foundation for several great products including the bottles, packets, dried wolfberries, Nitro®, and Zyng™.

# NINGXIA NITRO®

*Usage Ideas for Nitro®:*

- Afternoon pick-me-up
- Pre-workout
- Pre-interview
- Pre-test
- Pre-meeting
- Pre-presentation

Use this anytime there is a need for added mental clarity!

Here is what the makers say about this magical drink shot! "When you need a midday boost, it's easy to reach for things like soda and energy drinks. Skip the sugary solution and reboot with an option from Young Living. With NingXia Nitro®, you'll get a quick pick-me-up without the sugar or caffeine overload. Infused with essential oils, botanical extracts, D-ribose, Korean ginseng, and green tea extract, NingXia Nitro supports alertness, as well as cognitive and physical fitness.* A great support for body and mind wellness, use NingXia Nitro for running, weightlifting, or getting through your afternoon slump. The naturally occurring caffeine in Young Living's NingXia Nitro supports normal energy levels and alertness to help you with a busy day or a tough workout.* Stash Nitro wherever you need it! The small, convenient packaging makes it a great addition to your office desk, gym bag, or purse. Each box contains 14 20-ml tubes." ~ Young Living

INGREDIENTS
**Proprietary Nitro™ Energy blend:** D-Ribose, Green tea extract, Mulberry leaf extract, Korean ginseng extract, Choline (as Choline bitartrate)
**Proprietary Nitro Alert™ oil blend:** Vanilla absolute oil, Chocolate oil, Yerba mate oil, Spearmint oil, Peppermint oil, Nutmeg oil, Black Pepper oil, Wolfberry seed oil. Other Ingredients: Purified water, Nitro juice blend concentrate: (Cherry, Kiwi, Blueberry, Acerola, Billberry, Black currant, Raspberry, Strawberry, Cranberry), Coconut nectar, Natural flavors, Pectin, Xanthan gum

## NINGXIA ZYNG™

Forget those "really REALLY bad for you" energy drinks and sodas! Who needs a heart attack at 35? Not me! NingXia Zyng™ replaces all that yuck with something actually healthful for you! Here is what Young Living has to say about this great tasting energy drink:

"A hydrating splash of essential oil-infused goodness, NingXia Zyng™ uses the same whole-fruit wolfberry puree found in our popular superfruit supplement, NingXia Red®. We add sparkling water, pear and blackberry juices, and a hint of Lime and Black Pepper essential oils for a dynamic, unique taste. You'll enjoy a refreshing boost that's full of flavor without artificial flavors and preservatives. With natural flavors and sweeteners, white tea extract, and added vitamins, NingXia Zyng delivers 35 mg of naturally occurring caffeine and only 35 calories per can, making it a sweet, guilt-free boost for your early morning, long afternoon, or anytime you need a little Zyng!"

INGREDIENTS: Carbonated water, Evaporated cane sugar, Pear juice concentrate, Wolfberry (Lycium barbarum) puree, Citric acid, Blackberry juice concentrate, Natural flavor, White tea leaf extract, Stevia rebaudiana leaf extract, D-calcium pantothenate, Niacinamide, Black Pepper (Piper nigrum) fruit oil, Lime (Citrus latifolia) peel oil, D-alpha-tocopherol acetate, Pyridoxine hydrochloride, Retinyl palmitate.

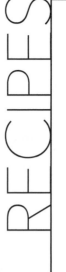

RECIPES

USAGE IDEAS

Ditch your morning coffee and opt for a much healthier alternative. Create a NingXia® BOMB!

Directions:

In a tall glass pour 2 ounces of NingXia Red®, add 1 NingXia Nitro® tube, and one can of NingXia Zyng™. Spike your drink with a drop of Thieves Vitality™, Tangerine Vitality™, or any oil of your choice.

**LESSON #28**

## *SUPPLEMENTS THAT WORK*

I love whole food nutrition and getting as much from what God has provided as possible. The reality is, the food sources we currently have access to are very different from those our grandparents or even parents grew up consuming. We have massively depleted our soils but more importantly, even if you are able to get organic farmer's market type produce and proteins, they are usually picked far before they should be. Did you know most produce is picked about 2 weeks before it is ripe? Did you also know that often the most vital phytonutrients are developed during the last few days of ripening?

It is unfortunate, but the reality is, we do not get the right vitamins and minerals in the normal food sources we eat. Supplementation is a great way to go, but sadly most supplements are synthetic or so isolated that your body does not know what to do with them so you end up having them go in one end only to go out the other without even getting into your system to be used. The act of something going into your body and your body using it is called the "bioavailability" of the item you are consuming.

I am not a fan of about 90% of the market's supplements for this reason alone. You are simply peeing and pooping your money right down the toilet. Not good... not good at all! It is why I absolutely love Young Living! I'll be honest with you, it took many years for me to even try their supplements because I was so skeptical. But OH MY! ... MY, OH MY! I am so impressed! You think oils are exciting?... Try these supplements! I saved supplements for last because there is a lot to cover. I will just be tickling the top of the iceberg so may I suggest you start looking into what you may need for yourself? You will love what you find. Not only are they bioavailable, but THEY WORK! Yay!

# NUTRITION THAT WORKS

## TARGETED SUPPLEMENTS

Young Living offers three types of nutritional supplements: Foundation, Cleansing, and Targeted.

### FOUNDATION NUTRITION

Noted by the blue label bottles, these are the vitamins and minerals that support a healthy diet. Young Living's vitamin supplement solutions feature food sourced vitamins and minerals that are bioavailable, meaning they will enter into your body correctly and be used by your body. They contain an infusion of essential oils, which have been proven to help them become even more bioavailable to support your needs.

### CLEANSING NUTRITION

Noted by the green label bottles, these are specifically designed to support the gastrointestinal tract. Complete with enzymes, probiotics, and specifically formulated products, these supplements help to support proper digestion for greater health and wellness!

### TARGETED NUTRITION

Noted by the orange label bottles, these are formulated with specific ingredients including powerful Essential Oils to support specific nutritional needs. These supplements target everything from enzyme support and joint health, to heart, brain, and digestive support.

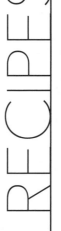

RECIPES

DIFFUSER RECIPE

I love being in nature! One of my favorite smells is when I am on a hike in a forest and the mixed melodies of tree aromas fill the air! Those are Essential Oils you are smelling! Take the outdoors inside with this fun conifer blend diffuser recipe:

- 4 drops Lemon
- 4 drops NL Black Spruce™
- 2 drops Pine
- 2 drops Cypress

TOPICAL RECIPE

Sun-lovers:
I love spending time outdoors. Sometimes I forget how long I have been in the sun and end up just a tad more pink than expected. A great way to cool your skin is to get a 4 ounce spray bottle and add about 1 drop of Lavender per ounce of water. Shake it up and spray it all over your skin.

# FOUNDATION NUTRITION *(BLUE LABELS)*

Foundation Nutrition, which are noted by the blue label bottles, are the vitamins and minerals that support a healthy diet. Young Living's vitamin supplement solutions feature food sourced vitamins and minerals that are bioavailable, meaning they will enter into your body correctly and be used by your body. They contain an infusion of Essential Oils, which have been proven to help them become even more bioavailable to support your needs.

## *MASTER FORMULA™ (FOUNDATION)*

If you want to choose an "All Star" for daily supplementation, Master Formula™ would be the winner. It is a three part daily supplement designed to support your full health spectrum. Young Living states, "Master Formula is a full spectrum, multinutrient complex, providing premium vitamins, minerals, and food-based nutriment to support general health and well-being. By utilizing a Synergistic Suspension Isolation process – SSI Technology – ingredients are delivered in three distinct delivery forms. Collectively, these ingredients provide a premium, synergistic complex to support your body.*"

### *BENEFITS*
- Naturally supports general health and well-being for the body
- Gut flora supporting prebiotics
- Ingredients help neutralize free radicals in the body
- Includes antioxidants, vitamins, minerals, and food-based nutriment
- Pre-packaged sachets are convenient to take your vitamins on the go
- SSI Technology delivers ingredients in 3 forms chosen for their complementary properties

### *MICRONIZED NUTRIENT CAPSULE*
This capsule supports the body naturally through lycopene, wolfberry powder, and citrus bioflavonoids. The capsule also contains Orgen-B's®, which is a blend of certified organic guava, mango, and lemon extracts for a perfect synergy of B vitamins and chelated minerals. It contains 100% natural vitamin B1, B2, B3, B5, B6, and B9. Orgen Family® states, "B-vitamins help critically with a range of normal body functions, from cellular growth to metabolism. Vitamin B3, also known as Niacin, helps in metabolism of glucose and fat. Vitamin B6, also known as pyridoxine, dominates the metabolism of amino acids and lipids. Vitamin B9 acts as a co-enzyme in the form of folates that aids the production of red blood cells."

### PHYTO-CAPLET

Contains trace minerals and gut flora-supporting prebiotics. Phyto-caplet also contains Spectra™, a powerful antioxidant that contains fruit, veggie, and herb extracts with Vitamin C. FutureCeuticals, Inc. states, "Spectra™ represents the latest evolution in the fight against potentially-damaging free radicals. For the first time anywhere, the biological effects of a natural supplement on the changes of oxidative and nitrosative stress markers, as well as cellular metabolic activity, have been clinically observed in the human body. Exclusively available from FutureCeuticals, Spectra™ has been reported to decrease ROS, increase cellular oxygen consumption in blood and mitochondria, decrease extracellular $H_2O_2$, and reduce TNFa-induced inflammatory response in humans."

### LIQUID VITAMIN CAPSULE

Contains Cardamom, Clove, Fennel, and Ginger essentials oils. The Liquid Vitamin Capsule also contains turmeric root oil, a powerfully oxygenating oil that supports overall health. This capsule contains fat soluble vitamins A, E, K, and a vegan sourced vitamin D3. These all provide excellent antioxidant support.

## MINERAL ESSENCE™ (FOUNDATION)

We often find ourselves depleted of the vital minerals we need every day. This powerful, fully balanced mineral tincture is the perfect way to supplement our growing mineral needs. Shake this well before you use. You can add the 5mLs needed to five 00 capsules or simply add it to 4-8 ounces of water. Young Living states, "Mineral Essence™ is a balanced, full-spectrum ionic mineral complex enhanced with essential oils. According to two time Nobel Prize winner Linus Pauling PhD. "You can trace every sickness, every disease, and every ailment to a mineral deficiency." Ionic minerals are the most fully and quickly absorbed form of minerals available."

*\*These statements have not been evaluated by the Food and Drug Administration. This product is not intended to diagnose, cure, treat, or prevent any disease.*

## LIFE 9™ (FOUNDATION)

Oh for the love of Life 9™! Have you ever gone to those health food stores and stood there like a deer in headlights looking at all the probiotics? Which one? This or that? I have tried so many your head would spin. Enter Life 9™. It is a little different than your garden variety probiotic. It has 9 strains to get you full-spectrum support, but what is interesting is that the best time to take it is at night just before bed. You take this without any other supplement. The very last thing at night. Then it goes to work. All those beautiful healthy bacteria helping support your beautiful gut! Seriously though, it is a beautiful thing to have a healthy gut. They say that 85% of all our issues stem from gut issues. So let's clean up our gut with Life 9™ probiotic!

Young Living states, "Life 9™ is a proprietary, high-potency probiotic that combines 17 billion live cultures from 9 beneficial bacteria strains that promotes healthy digestion, supports gut health, and helps maintain normal intestinal function for overall support of a healthy immune system.*
Life 9 is specially designed with special delayed-release capsules, a dual-sorbent desiccant, and a special bottle and cap that ensure your Life 9 stays fresh and effective. Each bottle contains 30 capsules, making it easy to use this helpful supplement daily."

Life 9™ includes 9 probiotic strains for full-spectrum gut support:

- Lactobacillus acidophilus
- Bifidobacterium lactis
- Lactobacillus plantarum
- Lactobacillus rhamnosus
- Lactobacillus salivarius
- Streptococcus thermophilus
- Bifidobacterium breve
- Bifidobacterium bifidum
- Bifidobacterium longum

*These statements have not been evaluated by the Food and Drug Administration. This product is not intended to diagnose, cure, treat, or prevent any disease.

## OMEGAGIZE3™ (FOUNDATION)

There are so many fish oil omega-3 fatty acid supplements you can choose from, but Young Living has far exceeded the all the others with OmegaGize3™! OmegaGize3™ is a core omega 3 supplement infused with an essential oil blend. Many of the Young Living supplements are infused with essential oils. Essential oils, when taken internally, can support health in a myriad of ways. Studies have shown that when infused with essential oils, the nutrients in the supplements become more bioavailable.

Young Living states, "OmegaGize3™ combines the power of three core daily supplements-omega 3 fatty acids, vitamin D-3, and CoQ10 (ubiquinone). These supplements combine with our proprietary enhancement essential oil blend to create an omega-3, DHA-rich fish oil supplement that may support general wellness. Used daily these ingredients work synergistically to support normal brain, heart, eye, and joint health.*"

## SUPER B™ (FOUNDATION)

Low on B vitamins? We've got you covered...all eight B vitamins! That is why it is called SUPER B™! Some of us need B vitamins every single day because our bodies are no longer storing them properly. B vitamins help keep our cells metabolizing correctly. They are water soluble and generally speaking are helpful with normal energy levels.

Young Living states, "Super B is a comprehensive vitamin complex containing all eight essential, energy-boosting B vitamins (B1, B2, B3, B5, B6, B7, B9, and B12). Recently reformulated, it now Features Orgen-FA®*, a natural folate source derived from lemon peels, and methylcobalamin, a more bioavailable source of B12. Combined with Nutmeg essential oil and bioavailable chelated minerals such as magnesium, manganese, selenium, and zinc, Super B not only assists in maintaining healthy energy levels, but it also supports mood and cardiovascular and cognitive function.* B vitamins are essential to our health and well-being, and each B vitamin performs a unique and separate function in the body. Unfortunately, they must be replenished daily, as they are not stored in the body."

*These statements have not been evaluated by the Food and Drug Administration. This product is not intended to diagnose, cure, treat, or prevent any disease.*

# CLEANSING NUTRITION *(GREEN LABELS)*

Cleansing Nutrition, noted by the green label bottles, are specifically designed to support the gastrointestinal tract. Complete with enzymes, probiotics, and specifically formulated nutrients, these supplements help to support digestion for greater health and wellness!

## COMFORTONE® (CLEANSING)

ComforTone® is the perfect supplement to support your stomach, digestion, liver, and gallbladder. Young Living states, "ComforTone® (capsules) is an effective combination of herbs and essential oils that support the health of the digestive system by eliminating residues from the colon and enhancing its natural ability to function optimally.* Because it supports normal peristalsis (the wave-like contractions that move food through the intestines), ComforTone is ideal for strengthening the system that delivers nutrients to the rest of the body.* It also contains ingredients that are beneficial to liver, gallbladder, and stomach health.*"

## ICP™ (CLEANSING)

ICP™ is Young Living's intestinal cleanse protocol.* Young Living states, "ICP™ helps keep your colon clean with an advanced mix of fibers that scour out residues.* A healthy digestive system is important for the proper functioning of all other systems because it absorbs nutrients that are used throughout the body. ICP provides ingredients such as psyllium, oat bran, and flax and fennel seeds to form a combination of soluble and insoluble fibers. Enhanced with a special blend of essential oils, the fibers work to decrease the buildup of wastes, improve nutrient absorption, and help maintain a healthy heart.* ICP provides two grams of dietary fiber, one gram of soluble fiber, and one gram of insoluble fiber per serving."

## JUVAPOWER® (CLEANSING)

JuvaPower® is the supplement to take when you need extra help with alkalizing your body. Young Living states, "JuvaPower® is a high antioxidant vegetable powder complex and is one of the richest sources of acid-binding foods. JuvaPower is rich in liver-supporting nutrients and has intestinal cleansing benefits.*"

*These statements have not been evaluated by the Food and Drug Administration. This product is not intended to diagnose, cure, treat, or prevent any disease.*

## JUVATONE® (CLEANSING)

JuvanTone® supports those who tend to eat more animal protein. Young Living states, "JuvaTone® is a powerful herbal complex designed to promote healthy liver function.* It is an excellent source of choline, a nutrient that is vital for proper liver function and necessary for those with high protein diets. JuvaTone also contains inositol and dl-methionine, which help with the body's normal excretion functions.* Methionine also helps recycle glutathione, a natural antioxidant crucial for normal liver function.* Other ingredients include Oregon grape root, a source of the liver-supporting compound berberine, and therapeutic-grade essential oils to enhance overall effectiveness.*"

## MULTIGREENS™ (CLEANSING)

MultiGreens™ is the perfect daily pairing to NingXia Red® for overall health support. Young Living states, "MultiGreens™ is a nutritious chlorophyll formula designed to boost vitality by working with the glandular, nervous, and circulatory systems.* MultiGreens is made with spirulina, alfalfa sprouts, barley grass, bee pollen, eleuthero, Pacific kelp, and therapeutic-grade essential oils."

Recommended usage: If you have a slow metabolism, take 3 capsules two times daily. If you have a fast metabolism, take 4 capsules once or twice daily. Best taken 1 hour before meals. For stomach sensitivity, take with meals.

## PARAFREE™ (CLEANSING)

Have you heard all the hype on the internet? Young Living has you covered. Young Living states, "ParaFree™ is formulated with an advanced blend of some of the strongest essential oils studied for their cleansing abilities.* This formula also includes the added benefits of sesame seed oil and olive oil."

## REHEMOGEN™ (CLEANSING)

Rehemogen™ supports healthy blood and detoxification. Young Living states, "Rehemogen™ contains Cascara sagrada, red clover, poke root, prickly ash bark, and burdock root, which have been his-torically used for their cleansing and building properties. Rehemogen is also formulated with essential oils to enhance digestion.*"

*These statements have not been evaluated by the Food and Drug Administration. This product is not intended to diagnose, cure, treat, or prevent any disease.*

# TARGETED NUTRITION *(ORANGE LABELS)*

Targeted Nutrition, which are noted by the orange label bottles, are formulated with specific ingredients including powerful Essential Oils to support specific nutritional needs. These supplements target everything from enzyme support and joint health, to heart, brain, and digestive support.

## AGILEASE™ (TARGETED)

This delightful little gem in the supplement lineup is no joke! If you need a little (or a lot) of extra help with healthy mobility, then AgilEase™ is the one for you! Young Living states, "Especially beneficial for athletes, as well as middle-aged and elderly people who may experience a natural, acute inflammation response in their joints after exercise, AgilEase™ is a joint health supplement that's perfect for healthy individuals who are looking to gain greater mobility and flexibility through the reduction of inflammation. We used unique and powerful ingredients such as frankincense powder, UC-II undenatured collagen, hyaluronic acid, calcium fructoborate, and a specially formulated proprietary essential oil blend of Wintergreen, Copaiba, Clove, and Northern Lights Black Spruce—oils that are known for their joint health benefits. Take AgilEase to support joint health or as a preventative measure to protect joint and cartilage health."

### BENEFITS
- Supports and protects joint and cartilage health*
- Beneficial for athletes and active individuals of all ages who want to support and protect their joints and cartilage*
- Perfect companion to an active lifestyle, promoting healthy joint function and supporting cartilage health*
- Supports the body's response to acute inflammation in healthy individuals*
- Helps support healthy joint flexibility and mobility*
- Formulated with ingredients and essential oils for healthy joint support*
- Helps ease acute joint discomfort to improve quality of life*

*These statements have not been evaluated by the Food and Drug Administration. This product is not intended to diagnose, cure, treat, or prevent any disease.*

## ALKALIME® (TARGETED)

AlkaLime® is a must for most people. It helps maintain the proper pH balance in the body. Young Living states, "AlkaLime® is a precisely-balanced alkaline mineral complex formulated to neutralize acidity and maintain desirable pH levels in the body. Infused with Lemon and Lime essential oils and organic whole lemon powder, AlkaLime also features enhanced effervescence and biochemic cell salts for increased effectiveness. A balanced pH is thought to play an important role in maintaining overall health and vigor."

### BENEFITS
- Absorbed easily and quickly by the body
- Effervescent formula starts working right away to soothe the occasional upset stomach
- Gentle on the stomach
- Helps maintain optimal pH in the stomach
- Free of artificial colors, flavors, or sweeteners, and formulated with nine biochemical mineral cell salts, the refreshing taste of Lemon and Lime essential oils, and organic lemon powder
- Comes in convenient, single-serve stick packs

## ALLERZYME™ (TARGETED)

Allerzyme™ to the rescue! Young Living states, "Allerzyme™ is a vegetarian enzyme complex that promotes digestion.* For the relief of occasional symptoms such as fullness, pressure, bloating, gas, pain, and/or minor cramping that may occur after eating."

## BLM™ (TARGETED)

BLM™ stands for bones, ligaments, and muscles. Young Living states, "BLM™ supports normal bone and joint health.* This formula combines powerful natural ingredients, such as type II collagen, MSM, glucosamine sulfate, and manganese citrate, enhanced with therapeutic-grade essential oils. These ingredients have been shown to support healthy cell function and encourage joint health and fluid movement.*"

*These statements have not been evaluated by the Food and Drug Administration. This product is not intended to diagnose, cure, treat, or prevent any disease.*

## AMINOWISE™ (TARGETED)

Aminowise™ is one of those special necessities for those of us who love to get in a good hard workout. You can drink this during your workout or directly after to help your body flush lactic acid buildup. Your body will be so happy you added this to your workout! I promise, your cells will smile!

Young Living states, "Optimize your workout recovery with the triple-targeted formula of AminoWise™. It uses three blends for one powerful result: The Muscle Performance blend aids muscle building and repair, the Recovery blend helps reduce muscle fatigue, and the Hydration Mineral blend replenishes important minerals lost during exercise. Simply mix 1 scoop with water and drink immediately after your workout to ensure that you're getting the most out of your hard work. AminoWise was developed and formulated to fill a need within the nutritional product line as a during and after-workout replenishing boost for the muscles. With a hydrating blend of minerals that are lost during exercise and with no added sugars, artificial sweeteners, preservatives, or artificial colors or flavors, AminoWise is a standout in the field of workout supplementation."

### BENEFITS
- A synergistic complex of amino acids and antioxidants that helps with fatigue and enhances muscle recovery during and after exercise
- A complex of antioxidants and minerals formulated to help reduce lactic acid induced by exercise
- Formulated to aid in reducing muscle fatigue
- Helps support the muscles during and after exercise to enhance recovery and performance
- Helps support the production of nitric oxide, which can improve vascular blood flow
- Contains branched chain amino acids, which have been shown to aid in preventing muscle catabolism from exercise
- Formulated to support hydration by replenishing important minerals lost during exercise
- Good source of vitamin E and zinc
- Formulated with wolfberry powder
- Flavored with Lemon and Lime Essential Oils
- No preservatives, synthetic colors, or artificial flavors
- No added sugar or artificial sweeteners

*These statements have not been evaluated by the Food and Drug Administration. This product is not intended to diagnose, cure, treat, or prevent any disease.*

## *CORTISTOP® (TARGETED)*

CortiStop® is a favorite of those who need a little help with the jitters. When life is coming at you from all sides, this is the thing to take right in the morning. Men can use it too, even though Young Living mentions it is for women. Young Living states, "CortiStop® Women's is a proprietary dietary supplement designed to help the body maintain its natural balance and harmony.* When under stress, the body produces cortisol. When cortisol is produced too frequently, it can have negative health consequences such as feelings of fatigue, difficulty maintaining healthy weight, and difficulty maintaining optimal health of cardiovascular systems. CortiStop supports the glandular systems of women.*"

## *DETOXZYME® (TARGETED)*

Detoxzyme® is an enzyme powerhouse to help you cleanse your system. Young Living states, "Detoxzyme® combines a myriad of powerful enzymes that complete digestion, help detoxify, and promote cleansing.* The ingredients in Detoxzyme also work with the body to support normal function of the digestive system, which is essential for maintaining and building health.*"

## *ENDOGIZE™ (TARGETED)*

Our endocrine system is what drives us. It is all of our hormones. Supporting the endocrine system is an important part of being the most healthy version of you! Young Living states, "EndoGize is especially formulated to support a healthy and balanced endocrine system in women.*"

## *ESSENTIALZYME™ (TARGETED)*

Essentialzyme™ helps support our crazy fluctuating diets by providing the essential enzymes needed to support digestion. Young Living states, "Essentialzyme™ is a bilayered, multienzyme complex caplet specially formulated to support and balance digestive health and to stimulate overall enzyme activity to combat the modern diet. Essentialzyme contains tarragon, peppermint, anise, fennel, and clove essential oils to improve overall enzyme activity, and support healthy pancreatic function."

*\*These statements have not been evaluated by the Food and Drug Administration. This product is not intended to diagnose, cure, treat, or prevent any disease.*

## ESSENTIALZYMES-4™ (TARGETED)

Essentialzymes-4™ helps support proper nutrient absorption. Young Living states, "Essentialzymes-4 is a multi-spectrum enzyme complex specially formulated to aid the critically needed digestion of dietary fats, proteins, fiber, and carbohydrates commonly found in the modern processed diet. The dual time-release technology releases the animal- and plant-based enzymes at separate times within the digestive tract, allowing for optimal nutrient absorption."

## FEMIGEN™ (TARGETED)

Femigen™ supports a healthy female reproductive system. Young Living states, "FemiGen™ capsules were formulated with herbs and amino acids designed to balance and support the female reproductive system from youth through menopause.* FemiGen combines whole food herbs like wild yam, damiana, and dong quai, along with synergistic amino acids and select essential oils to supply nutrition that is supportive of the special needs of the female systems.*

## IMMUPRO™ (TARGETED)

Strengthens my immune system and helps me fall asleep faster? Sign me up! One chewable tablet of ImmuPro™ about 30 minutes before bedtime and you are all set. It has just the right amount of non-habit forming melatonin, because it is from a natural source, to help you drift off to dreamland and then it gets to work with its amazing ability to fight all that oxidative stress that you built up during the day.

Young Living states, "ImmuPro™ has been specially formulated to provide exceptional immune system support when combined with a healthy lifestyle and adequate sleep to support the body's needs.* This power-packed formula combines naturally-derived immune-supporting NingXia wolfberry polysaccharides with a unique blend of reishi, maitake, and agaricus blazei mushroom powders to deliver powerful antioxidant activity to help reduce the damaging effects of oxidative stress from free radicals.* ImmuPro provides zinc and selenium for proper immune function* along with other chelated minerals which emerging science suggests are more easily absorbed by the body. It also delivers melatonin which encourages restful sleep by promoting the body's natural sleep rhythm.* With non-GMO dextrose instead of fructose and more Orange essential oil than ever, this formula delivers more of what you want and less of what you don't! This delicious fruit-flavored chewable supplement also has the same great wolfberry flavor but with a new crunchy texture."

*These statements have not been evaluated by the Food and Drug Administration. This product is not intended to diagnose, cure, treat, or prevent any disease.*

## K & B™ TINCTURE (TARGETED)

K & B™ is a must for renal system support. Young Living states, "K & B™ is formulated to nutritionally support normal kidney and bladder health.* It contains extracts of juniper berries, which enhance the body's efforts to maintain proper fluid balance; parsley, which supports kidney and bladder function and aids overall urinary health; and urva ursi, which supports both urinary and digestive system health.* K & B is enhanced with therapeutic-grade essential oils."

## MEGACAL™ (TARGETED)

MegaCal™ is a powdered formula to be mixed with water or juice for proper calcium absorbtion. Young Living states, "MegaCal™ is a wonderful source of calcium, magnesium, manganese, and vitamin C. MegaCal supports normal bone and vascular health as well as normal nerve function and contains 207 mg of calcium and 188 mg of magnesium per serving.*"

## MINDWISE™ AND MINDWISE™ SACHETS (TARGETED)

Help get your mind functioning back to its optimal performance! Young Living states, "Support normal cardiovascular health and cognitive health with the fruity, nutty flavor of MindWise™! With a vegetarian oil made from cold-pressed sacha inchi seeds harvested from the Peruvian Amazon and other medium-chain triglyceride oils, MindWise has a high proportion of unsaturated fatty acids and omega-3 fatty acids. Plus, it uses a combination of fruit juices and extracts, turmeric, and pure essential oils to create a heart and brain function supplement with a taste you'll love! MindWise also includes our proprietary memory function blend made with bioidentical CoQ10, ALCAR, and GPC—ingredients that have been studied for their unique benefits. With generous amounts of vitamin D3, this premium supplement is equipped to support normal brain function and overall cognitive and cardiovascular health.*"

### BENEFITS
- Supports normal brain and heart function*
- Contains a high proportion of unsaturated fatty acids and omega-3 fatty acids
- Includes beneficial GPC, ALCAR, and bioidentical CoQ10*
- Supports heart health by replenishing the body with CoQ10*
- Features an improved, smoother texture
- Includes no added preservatives
- Formulated with turmeric

*These statements have not been evaluated by the Food and Drug Administration. This product is not intended to diagnose, cure, treat, or prevent any disease.*

## PD 80/20™ (TARGETED)

PD 80/20™ has the proper balance of 80% Pregnenolone to 20% Dehydroepiandrosterone (DHEA) to help support your hormones. Young Living states, "PD 80/20™ is a dietary supplement formulated to help maximize internal health and support the endocrine system.* It contains pregnenolone and DHEA, two substances produced naturally by the body that decline with age. Pregnenolone is the key precursor for the body's production of estrogen, DHEA, and progesterone, and it also has an impact on mental acuity and memory.* DHEA is involved in maintaining the health of the cardiovascular and immune systems.*"

## POWERGIZE™ (TARGETED)

A favorite among athletes, Powergize™ can be utilized by any adult wishing to boost their physical game. Young Living states, "Inspire your inner athlete with PowerGize™! This supplement—infused with Blue Spruce, Goldenrod, and Cassia essential oils—is specially formulated to help individuals of all ages boost stamina and performance.* With botanicals from around the world, PowerGize helps sustain energy levels, strength, mental and physical vibrancy, and vitality when used in addition to physical activity.* PowerGize is also formulated with KSM-66, a premium ashwagandha root extract, which is touted for its properties that support immunity, mental clarity, concentration, and alertness. Its custom formula helps support the male reproductive system.*"

## PROSTATE HEALTH™ (TARGETED)

Specifically formulated for men, Prostate Health™ targets key elements to support the prostate. Young Living states, "Prostate Health is uniquely formulated for men concerned with supporting the male glandular system and maintaining healthy, normal prostate function. Prostate Health is an essential oil supplement featuring powerful saw palmetto and pumpkin seed oil—ingredients known for their support of a healthy prostate gland. A proprietary blend of pure geranium, fennel, myrtle, lavender, and peppermint essential oils provides the body with key components. The benefits of liquid capsules include a targeted release for ideal absorption and minimal aftertaste. For maximum benefit, Prostate Health should be taken consistently over time."

*These statements have not been evaluated by the Food and Drug Administration. This product is not intended to diagnose, cure, treat, or prevent any disease.*

## SULFURZYME® (TARGETED)

Sulfur is responsible for vital amino acids in our body to support healthy cells, skin, hormones, and enzymes. Young Living states, "Sulfurzyme® combines wolfberry with MSM, a naturally occurring organic form of dietary sulfur needed by our bodies every day to maintain the structure of proteins, protect cells and cell membranes, replenish the connections between cells, and preserve the molecular framework of connective tissue.* MSM also supports the immune system, the liver, circulation, and proper intestinal function and works to scavenge free radicals.* Wolfberries contain minerals and coenzymes that support the assimilation and metabolism of sulfur."

## SUPER CAL PLUS™ (TARGETED)

Start your morning off with supporting those bones! Eat a little something with these because it needs a little fat to get into your system. Even just a handful of nuts is good. This is not your mother's calcium supplement. Oh no! They are far better and so much more bioavailable. You will absolutely love these. They should become a part of your daily regimen for sure. Here is what Young Living says about them:

"There are plenty of calcium supplements you can choose from, but Super Cal Plus™ was created to offer more than just calcium and minerals—it is a true bone-health supplement. With a synergistic blend of bioavailable calcium, magnesium, vitamins D and K, and other trace minerals, Super Cal Plus supports the structure, integrity, and density of bones and teeth. Plus, adequate calcium and vitamin D throughout life as part of a well-balanced diet may reduce the risk of osteoporosis.*

Using a marine mineral blend derived from red algae that's harvested off the coast of Iceland, Super Cal Plus™ harnesses the power of naturally derived ingredients to bring you the vital minerals found in the most complete bone-support supplements. This unique seaweed absorbs calcium, magnesium, and other trace minerals from ocean water, bringing them together to support overall bone health, including bone-density support. Super Cal Plus™ also includes a unique fermented polysaccharide

*These statements have not been evaluated by the Food and Drug Administration. This product is not intended to diagnose, cure, treat, or prevent any disease.*

complex to support bone resorption and formation. With these powerhouse ingredients, plus a special blend of handpicked essential oils, Super Cal Plus™ plays an important role in maintaining overall bone health to help you stay moving.*"

## BENEFITS

- Uses a synergistic blend of bioavailable calcium, magnesium, and other trace minerals derived from red algae harvested off the coast of Iceland
- Features a dual-action blend that helps maintain and support the structure, integrity, and density of bones*
- Promotes healthy bones by supporting the body's ability to resorb bone tissue (osteoclasts) and deposit new bone tissue (osteoblasts)*
- Provides an excellent source of calcium, magnesium, vitamin K, and vitamin D
- Helps support and contribute to the maintenance of healthy bones using calcium, magnesium, and a unique matrix of trace minerals*

## THYROMIN™ (TARGETED)

If your thyroid gets blamed often for your shortcomings, try supporting it with Thyromin™. This essential supplement is a great choice to support your metabolism and energy. Young Living states, "Thyromin™ is a special blend of porcine glandular extracts, herbs, amino acids, minerals, and therapeutic-grade essential oils in a perfectly balanced formula that maximizes nutritional support for healthy thyroid function.* The thyroid gland regulates body metabolism, energy, and body temperature."

# POWERHOUSE INGREDIENTS

*These statements have not been evaluated by the Food and Drug Administration. This product is not intended to diagnose, cure, treat, or prevent any disease.*

# SUPPLEMENT SCHEDULE & ALLERGY INFO

### TAKE ANYTIME

Agilease™
AminoWise™
Balance Complete™
ComforTone®
Inner Defense™
JuvaPower®
JuvaTone®
K & B™
Longevity™
Master Formula™
MegaCal™
MindWise™
Mineral Essence™
MultiGreens™
NingXia Nitro™
NingXia Red®
NingXia® Wolfberries
PD 80/20™
Powergize™
Prostate Health
Pure Protein Complete™
Rehemogen™
Slique® Bars
Slique® Essence
Slique® Gum
Slique® Tea
Sulfurzyme®
Super B™
Super C™
Super Cal Plus™

### BEFORE BREAKFAST

AlkaLime®
Allerzyme™
Cortistop®
Digest + Cleanse™
Essentialzyme™
ICP™
Inner Defense™
KidScents MightyVites™
NingXia Red®
OmegaGize³™
ParaFree™
Slique® CitraSlim™

### WITH FOOD

BLM™
EndoGize™
Essentialzymes-4™
Estro™
FemiGen™
JuvaPower®
KidScents MightyZyme™
Master Formula™
MegaCal™
MindWise™
MultiGreens™
Rehemogen ™
Slique® Tea
Super B™
Super C™
Super Cal Plus™

### BETWEEN MEALS

AlkaLime®
Detoxyme®
Digest + Cleanse™
Essentialzyme™
KidScents MightyVites™
Mineral Essence™
OmegaGize³™
ParaFree™
Slique® Bars
Slique® Essence
Slique® Gum
Slique® CitraSlim™
Sulfurzyme®

### AT BEDTIME

AlkaLime®
Detoxyme®
ICP™
ImmuPro™
Inner Defense™
Life 9™
MegaCal™
SleepEssence
Thyromin™

### OILS ONLY

Digest + Cleanse™
Inner Defense™
Longevity™
SleepEssence

### NOT VEGAN

Allerzyme™
BLM™
Inner Defense™
Longevity™
Master Formula™
MultiGreens™
OmegaGize™
Prostate Health™
Pure Protein™ Complete
Slique® Bars
Super C™
Super Cal Plus™
Thyromin™

### CONTAINS GLUTEN

Allerzyme™
Balance Complete™
Essentialzymes-4™
ICP™
JuvaPower®
KidScents MightyVites™
Master Formula™
MultiGreens™

### CONTAINS DAIRY

Allerzyme™
Balance Complete™
Pure Protein™ Complete
Super C™

### CONTAINS NUTS

MindWise™
Slique® Bars
Slique® CitraSlim™

# ESSENTIAL OIL SUPPLEMENTS

Young Living offers so many amazing oil-based supplements, it is easy to see why they are the best resource for foundation, cleansing, and targeted nutrition. In this section we will see how you can supplement your health through the use of pure essential oil supplements. It is no secret that Young Living is known for their amazing essential oils. The oils are what set their supplements apart from every other supplement on the market. Most supplements are infused with essential oils. These remarkable oils work in all sorts of ways to help support and promote better health.

## EO SUPPLEMENT: DIGEST + CLEANSE™ (CLEANSING)

Contains 12 drops total of Coconut carrier and pure essential oils.
Essential oils: Peppermint, Caraway, Lemon, Ginger, Fennel, and a small amount of Anise with virgin Coconut and fractionated Coconut carrier.

Digest + Cleanse™ is oh so helpful for those of us who have tummy troubles. It can become your best friend! I highly recommend having this in your stash and taking it on a regular basis. Young Living says, "Digest + Cleanse™ soothes gastrointestinal upset and supports healthy digestion.* Stress, overeating, and toxins can irritate the gastrointestinal system and cause cramps, gas, and nausea that interfere with the body's natural digestive and detox functions. Supplementing with Digest + Cleanse will soothe the bowel, prevent gas, and stimulate stomach secretions, thus aiding digestion.* Digest + Cleanse is formulated with clinically proven and time-tested essential oils that work synergistically to help prevent occasional indigestion and abdominal pain.* Precision Delivery softgels release in the intestines for optimal absorption and targeted relief and to help prevent aftertaste. This product can also be used in conjunction with any cleansing program, such as Young Living's 5-Day Nutritive Cleanse. Digest + Cleanse is part of the new Purely Oils line of premium essential oil supplements."

## EO SUPPLEMENT: INNER DEFENSE™ (FOUNDATION)

Contains 13 drops total of Coconut carrier and pure essential oils.
Essential oils: Clove, Lemon, Eucalyptus radiata, Rosemary, Cinnamon bark, Oregano, Thyme, and Lemongrass with virgin Coconut carrier.

Inner Defense™ is a beautiful immunity boosting essential oil supplement designed to help in several areas of health. Commonly referred to as a "terrain strengthener", Inner Defense is safe to consume daily, but can also be taken on days you are not feeling your best. The mix of Thieves® with added Oregano, Thyme, and Lemongrass make this an incredible health "bomb". Contrary to popular assumption, taking this daily will not upset the good gut flora. Oregano and the other oils in this capsule work in harmony with your gut helping to strengthen your terrain rather than beat it up. Young

*These statements have not been evaluated by the Food and Drug Administration. This product is not intended to diagnose, cure, treat, or prevent any disease.*

Living states, "Young Living's Inner Defense™ reinforces systemic defenses, creates unfriendly terrain for yeast/fungus, promotes healthy respiratory function, and contains potent essential oils like Oregano, Thyme, and Thieves® which are rich in thymol, carvacrol, and eugenol for immune support. The liquid softgels dissolve quickly for maximum results. Softgel capsule has been reformulated with fish gelatin to remove the need for carrageenan and bees wax used in the porcine gelatin based softgel."

## EO SUPPLEMENT: LONGEVITY™ (FOUNDATION)
Contains 14 drops total of Coconut carrier and pure essential oils.
Essential oils: Thye, Orange, Clove, and Frankincense with virgin Coconut and fractionated Coconut carrier.
Oh Longevity! These capsules are pre-mixed essential oil synergies ready to consume. The best part is they come in thick walled capsules that are designed to dissolve in your intestines rather than your stomach. This is important because getting oils into your intestines promotes better health than allowing your stomach acids to come in contact with the oils. While stomach acid is not a huge offense to oils, there are some added benefits to getting them into your intestines rather than your digestive system. Supporting your gut goes a long way to longevity!

Young Living states, "Longevity™ softgels are a potent, proprietary blend of fat-soluble antioxidants. Longevity blend should be taken daily to strengthen the body's systems to prevent the damaging effects of aging, diet, and the environment.* Enriched with the pure essential oils Thyme, Orange, and Frankincense, Longevity protects DHA levels, a nutrient that supports brain function and cardiovascular health, promotes healthy cell regeneration, and supports liver and immune function.* Longevity also contains clove oil, nature's strongest antioxidant, for ultra antioxidant support."

## EO SUPPLEMENT: SLEEPESSENCE (TARGETED)
Contains 12.8 drops total of Coconut carrier and pure essential oils with 3.2 mg Melatonin.
Essential oils: Lavender, Vetiver, Valerian, Tangerine, and Rue with virgin Coconut carrier and Melatonin.
This targeted essential oil supplement is a must if you need help in the sleep department. Young Living states, "SleepEssence contains four powerful Young Living Therapeutic Grade™ essential oils that have unique sleep-enhancing properties in a softgel vegetarian capsule for easy ingestion. Combining Lavender, Vetiver, Valerian, and Ruta Graveolens essential oils with the hormone melatonin—a well-known sleep aid—SleepEssence is a natural way to enable a full night's rest."

*These statements have not been evaluated by the Food and Drug Administration. This product is not intended to diagnose, cure, treat, or prevent any disease.*

# MEAL REPLACEMENT SUPPLEMENTS

Young Living offers one of the most comprehensive meal replacement and snack supplement lines on the market today. You could almost be fully covered with your NingXia Red® and these meal replacement options if necessary. The full weight management line called Slique® Complete is a proven way to support your weight-loss goals.

## BALANCE COMPLETE™ (FOUNDATION)

Balance Complete™ is a great way to support your Young Living 5-day cleanse. You replace your three daily meals with two scoops of Balance Complete™ mixed with 8-10 ounces of cold-water or milk. This makes a great once-daily meal replacement for health maintenance. If you are looking to help support weight management, simply replace two meals per day with Balance Complete™.

Young Living states, "Balance Complete™ is a super-food-based meal replacement that is both a powerful nutritive energizer and a cleanser. Offering the benefits of NingXia wolfberry powder, brown rice bran, barley grass, extra virgin coconut oil, aloe vera, cinnamon powder, and our premium whey protein blend, Balance Complete is high in fiber, high in protein, and contains the good fats, enzymes, vitamins, and minerals needed for a nutritionally dynamic meal. Balance Complete also features Young Living's proprietary V-Fiber™ blend, which supplies an amazing 11 grams of fiber per serving, absorbs toxins, and satisfies the appetite while balancing the body's essential requirements.*"

## PURE PROTEIN™ COMPLETE (TARGETED)

Pure Protein™ Complete shake mix comes in both vanilla and chocolate. The thing that impresses me most about this shake is that it keeps me full much longer than other meal replacement shakes. This is due to the fact that it contains five different proteins that your body processes at different rates. Here is what Young Living says about it:

Young Living states, "Pure Protein Complete is a comprehensive protein supplement that combines a proprietary 5-Protein Blend,

*These statements have not been evaluated by the Food and Drug Administration. This product is not intended to diagnose, cure, treat, or prevent any disease.*

amino acids, and ancient peat and apple extract to deliver 25 grams of protein per serving in two delicious flavors, Vanilla Spice and Chocolate Deluxe. Its foundation of cow and goat whey, pea protein, egg white protein, and organic hemp seed protein provide a full range of amino acids including: D-aspartic acid, Threonine, L-serine, Glutamic acid, Glycine, Alanine, Valine, Methionine, Isoleucine, Leucine, Tyrosine, Phenylalanine, Lysine, Histidine, Arginine, Proline, Hydroxyproline, Cystine, Tryptophan, and Cysteine. Along with a proprietary enzyme blend, these amino acids support overall protein utilization in the body. Ancient peat and apple extract, along with a powerful B-vitamin blend, complete the formula. Together they support ATP production, the energy currency of the body. This innovative formula makes Pure Protein Complete the perfect option for those looking for a high protein supplement that features a full range of amino acids."

## *BENEFITS*

- Excellent source of protein
- Optimal 5-Protein Blend
- Protein Boost
- Supports the body's need for protein
- Protein metabolism support
- elevATP or Ancient peat and Apple extract supports ATP production, the energy currency of the body
- Offers 25 grams of protein
- No trans fat
- rBGH-Free Whey
- Soy-Free
- High in Protein
- Supports muscular system
- Supports body in building lean muscle
- Supports ATP production
- Delivers amino acids
- Supports energy levels
- Post-workout muscle recovery
- Provides a full range of Amino Acids including: D-aspartic acid, Threonine, L-serine, Glutamic acid, Glycine, Alanine, Valine, Methionine, Isoleucine, Leucine, Tyrosine, Phenylalanine, Lysine, Histidine, Arginine, Proline, Hydroxyproline, Cystine, Tryptophan, and Cysteine

*\*These statements have not been evaluated by the Food and Drug Administration. This product is not intended to diagnose, cure, treat, or prevent any disease.*

## SLIQUE® SHAKE

Slique products are designed to help you maintain a healthy weight. The Slique system combines a meal replacement shake, snack bars, tea, gum and other items to help you reach your goals! This is a proven system and I highly recommend it!

Young Living says, "Slique® Shake is a complete meal replacement that provides quick, satisfying, and delicious nutrition. Formulated with Slique Essence essential oil blend, this shake may support healthy weight management when combined with regular exercise and a sensible diet.* In a convenient single-serving size packet, it's easy to slip into a purse or pocket for healthy eating on the go."

## SLIQUE™ BARS (REGULAR & CHOCOLATE COATED)

Young Living states, "Slique Bars dual-targeted satiety approach and medley of exotic fruits, nuts, and science creates the perfect functional, nutritious snack to help you feel fuller, longer. Members have always enjoyed Slique® Bars as a delicious weight-management tool that utilizes a dual-target approach to help manage satiety. Now this innovative bar is coated in delicious dark chocolate! To support any weight-management plan, Slique® Bars are loaded with exotic baru nuts and wholesome almonds, which promote satiety when combined with protein and fiber. We also use a potato skin extract that, when ingested, triggers the release of cholecystokinin in the body, increasing the duration of feelings of fullness. Slique® Bars deliver essential nutrients from a unique superfruit blend of goldenberries and wolfberries, plus pure Cinnamon, Vanilla, and Orange essential oils. This dual-target satiety approach and medley of exotic fruits, nuts, and potato skin extract create a nutritious, stimulant-free snack to help you feel fuller, longer."

### BENEFITS
- High in fiber
- Gluten-free
- No trans fat
- No preservatives
- Manages satiety
- Potato skin extract triggers the release of cholecystokinin (CCK) in the body, increasing the duration of feelings of fullness
- A mix of exotic nuts and berries, featuring baru nuts, goldenberries, and wolfberries, delivers delicious taste and promotes fullness when combined with protein and high levels of fiber
- A proprietary essential oil blend of Cinnamon, Vanilla, and Orange essential oils helps moderate cravings

## SLIQUE® CITRASLIM™

Young Living states, "Slique® CitraSlim™ is formulated with naturally derived ingredients to promote healthy weight management when combined with a balanced diet and regular exercise.* Slique CitraSlim also includes a proprietary citrus extract blend, which some studies suggest may help support the body in burning excess fat when used in conjunction with a healthy weight-management plan.* This polyphenolic mixture of flavonoids offers powerful antioxidants that are touted for their health benefits.* This blend may also support the release of free fatty acids, which help break down fat.* "

*ONCE-DAILY LIQUID CAPSULE:* The liquid capsule delivers pomegranate seed oil, Lemongrass, Lemon Myrtle, and Idaho Balsam Fir Essential Oils. This blend is high in citral, which is a constituent that may increase metabolic activity.*

*POWDER CAPSULES:* Three power-packed powder capsules contain a proprietary citrus extract blend, cinnamon powder, bitter orange extract, fenugreek seed, ocotea leaf extract, and a customized blend of enzymes and four Essential Oils: Ocotea, Cassia, Spearmint, and Fennel.

## SLIQUE® GUM

Young Living states, "Ancient travelers throughout the Middle East used raw frankincense resin for its nutritional content and ability to help control hunger. Slique® Gum offers those same benefits in a modern delivery system that helps control food cravings and improve oral health."

## SLIQUE® ESSENCE ESSENTIAL OIL

Young Living states, "Slique Essence combines Grapefruit, Tangerine, Lemon, Spearmint, and Ocotea with stevia extract in a unique blend that supports healthy weight management goals. These ingredients work together to help control hunger*, especially when used in conjunction with Slique Tea or the Slique Kit. The pleasant citrus combination of Grapefruit, Tangerine, and Lemon essential oils adds a flavorful and uplifting element to any day with the added support of spearmint that may help with digestion.* Ocotea essential oil adds an irresistible, cinnamon-like aroma to help control hunger, while stevia adds an all-natural sweetener that provides a pleasant taste with no added calories."

*\*These statements have not been evaluated by the Food and Drug Administration. This product is not intended to diagnose, cure, treat, or prevent any disease.*

**LESSON #29**

## ESSENTIAL REWARDS

Young Living truly honors their loyal customers. They want you to get the most out of their products so they have created a great loyalty incentive program called Essential Rewards (ER). ER is their easy automatic shipment program that allows you to order exactly what you want, when you want, hassle-free while getting up to 25% back in points to spend on products you want to try or already love. This course will help you see the benefits of this incredible program and how to sign up. You will also find easy suggestions for your first few orders so you can get the hang of it.

## BENEFITS OF ESSENTIAL REWARDS

### EASY MONTHLY SHIPMENTS
Your favorite products come every month or you can select different products each month.
Low minimum of only 50PV to stay active in ER!

### REDUCED SHIPPING
Shipping options start at just $5.99!

### EARN FREE PRODUCT
Earn points toward future purchases!
Months 1 to 3 get 10% back
Months 4 to 24 get 20% back
Months 25+ get 25% back
(1PV or point usually equals $1)

### EXCLUSIVE FREE BONUS OILS
Earn free exclusive oils at 100PV & 190PV levels.
Plus, get more free promos at 250PV and 300PV.

### EXCLUSIVE LOYALTY GIFTS
Earn gifts and get rewarded when you order for 3, 6, and 9 consecutive months. Plus, you'll get an exclusive Essential Reward blend at your 12th month!

### HASSLE FREE PROGRAM
Change your order, change your shipping date, or cancel Essential Rewards all together! You can use your points as soon as your second month that you've been enrolled.

## *HOW TO SIGN UP*

Follow these simple steps:

1. Log in to your wholesale membership account at www.youngliving.com under the Virtual Office.

2. Select Essential Rewards in the left bar menu.

3. Follow the instructions to sign up!

4. Select your monthly amount (minimum 50PV).

5. Sign up for PV assistant so your order never falls below your desired PV. You would not want to miss out on those promos!

6. If you have questions, you can call customer service at 800-371-3515.

Essential Rewards is something that just makes sense. What company gives you back up to 25%? I don't know of any. Plus it is so flexible that there really isn't a good reason NOT to be on Essential Rewards.

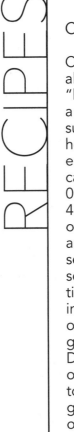

## CAPSULES

Capsules, also known as "bombs" are a great way to support your health. Get some empty veggie capsules in size 00. Use at least 4 drops of carrier oil to avoid any heartburn sensation. Create several at a time and store in your freezer or fridge in a glass container. Drip 1 drop each of the following, top off with grapeseed or olive oil, and take in the morning for no more than 5 days at a time.

FLUSHING: Vitality™ line Peppermint, Lemon, Grapefruit

ENERGY: Vitality™ line Black Pepper, Nutmeg, and Lemon

FOCUS: Vitality™ line Copaiba, Frankincense, and Lavender

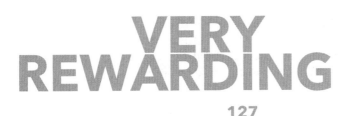

**LESSON #30**

# CONGRATS, YOU'VE FINISHED!

Congratulations! You've reached the finish line!
I am so proud of you for sticking through the full 30-day course!
Phew! It was a lot to take in! I encourage you to go back to
reread some or all of them. Below are a few extra resources
to learn more about the VITALITY Young Living Lifestyle.

# FACEBOOK RESOURCES

### THE HUMAN BODY AND ESSENTIAL OILS GROUP
**www.Facebook.com/groups/TheHumanBody**
Join The Human Body and Essential Oils, the largest online free
educational group lead by one Young Living educator, Jen O'Sullivan.
You get my shoot-from-the-hip, no-nonsense style of delivery, and
I am one of the only people who will tackle the truly difficult and
controversial subjects. I don't shy away from hype or helping people
overcome potential misunderstandings. I am a truth seeker and
while I am human and do make mistakes, my number one goal has
always been and will always be to dig up the truth and share it with
you. This is a completely free group that I post in often, so if you are
not in this group, get yourself in there ASAP! You won't regret it!

### JEN O'SULLIVAN'S AUTHOR PAGE
**www.Facebook.com/JenOSullivanAuthor**
My author page is a place where I provide content that you can
share in your own groups and pages. Just hit the "Share" button!

### SAVVY FACE GROUP
**www.Facebook.com/groups/SavvyFace**
Savvy Face is an online tutorial and forum group dedicated to educating
about the Savvy Minerals makeup line by Young Living with a plethora
of free learning tutorials. With over 40 video tutorials and tons of other
vital information, you will for sure want to join this group. Again, this
group is fully free! Yay! Make sure you check out the pinned post!

### IGNITE ACADEMY
**www.Facebook.com/groups/IgniteAcademy**
This is a group for serious learners. It is a study group and place
to get discount codes on the absolute best aromatherapy courses
there are from The New York Institute of Aromatic Studies.

# ONLINE RESOURCES

## INSTAGRAM
**@JenAuthor**
Instagram is another way to connect with me. I post snippets of videos I am doing and helpful tips. Feel free to follow me and tag me in your posts!

## YOUTUBE
**www.JensTips.com**
My YouTube channel contains shareable content for those not on Facebook. There are lots of informative videos that you can share with your friends!

# APP RESOURCES

There are two apps worth checking out.
**The EO Bar** app and the **Live Well with Young Living** app.

## THE EO BAR
The EO Bar app is the largest educational app for essential oils on the market. It's available on Android and Apple mobile devices. There is an exceptional amount of educational information in this app including over 300 recipes! Plus we are adding to it all the time. It is a one-time app purchase and then you get all the amazing updates for free as they happen. If you want to learn how to use oils best, get this app. By the way, this app was developed by over 500 Young Living distributors and 100 of them played a huge role in determining exactly how it looked and worked. We all wanted a better app, so this is literally the app Young Living distributors built! I am just honored to be a part of it all!

## LIVE WELL WITH YOUNG LIVING
Live Well with Young Living app is the easiest place to learn all about your Young Living Premium Starter Kit. It gives you an easy to follow Oils 101 basic course based on the country you choose. This is a great app to gift to new customers who are just starting out. You can easily switch between countries so you know how to share Essential Oils with friends around the world!

# PRINTED RESOURCES

## 31 OILS - EDUCATIONAL TOOLS
**www.31oils.com**
**www.facebook.com/31oils**
31 Oils, LLC is a company that produces and distributes my educational resources. They carry all my books at bulk pricing as well as some really amazing tools such as an Essential Oil Usage Guide brochure that showcases 55 of the most popular essential oils. There are several explanation cards offered such as The Premium Starter Kit, Essential Rewards (giving ideas for future orders), New Member Sign-up Info, and Starter Kit Challenge as well as several other really fun and informative tools. They ship quickly and most items ship Priority mail. Also, be sure to check out the Human Body and Essential Oils group on Facebook for special sale announcements.

## BOOKS!
**www.Amazon.com**
**www.31oils.com**
I have written several books over the years and my essential oil books have all been on the Amazon bestseller list! That is totally crazy to me! I am humbled and thankful for you all! You can view them on my Author page on Amazon or just type in my name and they should all come up. If you've ever wondered what order I would recommend reading them in, here you go:

- *The Essential Oil Truth: The Facts Without the Hype*

- *Vitality: The Young Living Lifestyle*

- *French Aromatherapy: Essential Oil Recipes and Usage Guide*

- *Live Well: Essential Oils for Wellness, Purpose, and Abundance*

- *Essential Oil Make & Takes: Over 60 DIY Projects and Recipes for the Perfect Class*

- *Essentially Driven: Young Living Essential Oils Business Handbook*

## FINAL THOUGHTS

If you haven't figured me out by now, I LOVE educating. Young Living is an astounding company that we all can stand behind because they go ahead of us making sure their products are the best available! Thank you for being on this journey with me and I look forward to seeing you online! The YL Family is something I never saw coming and I would never give it up for anything!

Young Living has changed my life in ways I cannot begin to explain. My gratitude for them, and also for you, has been an astounding blessing to me and my family! I had absolutely no clue what I was getting into when I started opening my big fat mouth about essential oils. Funny how life works!

What an honor! I love my Young Living family and will continue to give of myself as much as I possibly can! I love you all and wish the best life for you! The Lord has absolutely blessed me through you! Live well with VITALITY, my friend! Live Well!

**By the way, don't forget to join the VITALITY Book Club for additional free resources on Facebook at www.Facebook.com/groups/VitalityBook**

See you online!

~ Jen

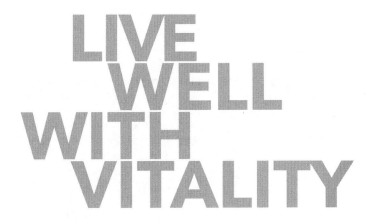

# "PRODUCTS FOR A PURPOSE"

~ D. Gary Young

This easy to use Young Living Product Price Guide is compiled so you can see all the products in one place. This book contains most of the products in the catalogue, but you will find some that were not mentioned, yet are still well loved! The cookware is simply, hands down the best you can buy. The other food items, like Einkorn and the NingXia Berry Syrup, will blow you away. The complete kid's and animal lines are a must for families of all sizes!

Please note, the prices are subject to change and the products offered often expand. Please always check with the official Young Living website for all the up-to-date information on their current prices and amazing products!

www.YoungLiving.com

PRODUCT PRICE GUIDE

# PREMIUM STARTER KITS

| Starter Kits | Item | WhSl | Retail | PV |
|---|---|---|---|---|
| EO PSK with Dewdrop Diffuser | 5463 | $160 | ($340) | 100PV |
| EO PSK with Desert Mist Diffuser | 22397 | $160 | ($340) | 100PV |
| EO PSK with Rainstone Diffuser | 5470 | $205 | ($486) | 100PV |
| EO PSK with Aria Diffuser | 5465 | $260 | ($561) | 100PV |
| Savvy Minerals PSK Cool 2 | 23830 | $150.00 | ($253) | 100PV |
| Savvy Minerals PSK Warm 2 | 23834 | $150.00 | ($253) | 100PV |
| Savvy Minerals PSK Dark 1 | 23832 | $150.00 | ($253) | 100PV |
| Savvy Minerals PSK Dark 4 | 23833 | $150.00 | ($253) | 100PV |
| NingXia Red PSK | 5467 | $170.00 | ($320) | 100PV |
| Thieves PSK | 5466 | $160.00 | ($310) | 100PV |

# SINGLES

| Essential Oil Singles | Item | WhSl | Retail | PV |
|---|---|---|---|---|
| Angelica 5 ml | 3078 | $45.00 | $59.21 | 45PV |
| Basil 15 ml | 3500 | $25.50 | $33.55 | 25.50PV |
| Bergamot 15 ml | 3503 | $27.75 | $36.51 | 27.75PV |
| Black Pepper 5 ml | 3611 | $19.25 | $25.33 | 19.25PV |
| Blue Cypress 5 ml | 3083 | $29.75 | $39.14 | 29.75PV |
| Blue Tansy 5 ml | 3084 | $94.75 | $124.67 | 94.75PV |
| Cardamom 5 ml | 3080 | $26.00 | $34.21 | 26PV |
| Carrot Seed 5 ml | 3081 | $22.25 | $29.28 | 22.25PV |
| Cedarwood 15 ml | 3509 | $11.50 | $15.13 | 11.50PV |
| Cinnamon Bark 5 ml | 3515 | $24.75 | $32.57 | 24.75PV |
| Cistus 5 ml | 3518 | $64.50 | $84.87 | 64.50PV |
| Citronella 15 ml | 3085 | $20.00 | $26.32 | 20PV |
| Clary Sage 15 ml | 3521 | $48.75 | $64.14 | 48.75PV |
| Clove 15 ml | 3524 | $15.75 | $20.72 | 15.75PV |
| Copaiba 15 ml | 3431 | $44.25 | $58.22 | 44.25PV |
| Coriander 5 ml | 3527 | $32.25 | $42.43 | 32.25PV |
| Cypress 15 ml | 3530 | $19.75 | $25.99 | 19.75PV |
| Dill 5 ml | 3536 | $16.25 | $21.38 | 16.25PV |
| Dorado Azul 5 ml | 3598 | $35.50 | $46.71 | 35.50PV |
| Elemi 15 ml | 3540 | $21.75 | $28.62 | 21.75PV |
| Eucalyptus Blue 5 ml | 3597 | $15.50 | $20.39 | 15.50PV |
| Eucalyptus Globulus 15 ml | 3539 | $14.75 | $19.41 | 14.75PV |
| Eucalyptus Radiata 15 ml | 3538 | $19.00 | $25.00 | 19PV |
| Fennel 15 ml | 3542 | $17.75 | $23.36 | 17.75PV |
| Frankincense 15 ml | 3548 | $75.50 | $99.34 | 75.50PV |
| Geranium 15 ml | 3554 | $42.50 | $55.92 | 42.50PV |
| German Chamomile 5 ml | 3086 | $37.50 | $49.34 | 37.50PV |
| Ginger 5 ml | 3557 | $13.50 | $17.76 | 13.50PV |
| Goldenrod 5 ml | 3562 | $15.75 | $20.72 | 15.75PV |
| Grapefruit 15 ml | 3560 | $17.25 | $22.70 | 17.25PV |
| Helichrysum 5 ml | 3563 | $87.50 | $115.13 | 87.50PV |
| Hinoki 5 ml | 3073 | $25.50 | $33.55 | 25.50PV |

| Essential Oil Singles (continued) | Item | WhSl | Retail | PV |
|---|---|---|---|---|
| Hyssop 5 ml | 3566 | $26.00 | $34.21 | 26PV |
| Idaho Balsam Fir 5 ml | 3314 | $26.75 | $35.20 | 26.75PV |
| Idaho Balsam Fir 15 ml | 3316 | $64.50 | $84.87 | 64.50PV |
| Idaho Blue Spruce 5 ml | 3093 | $29.50 | $38.82 | 29.50PV |
| Jade Lemon 5 ml | 4685 | $11.00 | $14.47 | 11PV |
| Jasmine 5 ml | 3569 | $78.75 | $103.62 | 78.75PV |
| Juniper 15 ml | 3572 | $34.50 | $45.39 | 34.50PV |
| Lavender 15 ml | 3575 | $24.25 | $31.91 | 24.25PV |
| Ledum 5 ml | 3579 | $64.50 | $84.87 | 64.50PV |
| Lemon 15 ml | 3578 | $11.50 | $15.13 | 11.50PV |
| Lemon Myrtle 5 ml | 3079 | $23.25 | $30.59 | 23.25PV |
| Lemongrass 15 ml | 3581 | $11.50 | $15.13 | 11.50PV |
| Lime 15 ml | 3074 | $12.50 | $16.45 | 12.50PV |
| Manuka 5 ml | 5322 | $36.75 | $48.36 | 36.75PV |
| Marjoram 15 ml | 3584 | $35.75 | $47.04 | 35.75PV |
| Mastrante 5 ml | 4686 | $26.50 | $34.87 | 26.50PV |
| Melaleuca Quinquenervia 15 ml | 3089 | $32.25 | $42.43 | 32.25PV |
| Melissa 5 ml | 3589 | $162.25 | $213.49 | 81PV |
| Mountain Savory 5 ml | 3590 | $25.50 | $33.55 | 25.50PV |
| Myrrh 15 ml | 3593 | $66.75 | $87.83 | 66.75PV |
| Neroli 5 ml | 3088 | $106.75 | $140.46 | 106.75PV |
| Northern Lights Black Spruce 5 ml | 5313 | $24.50 | $32.24 | 24.50PV |
| Northern Lights Black Spruce 15 ml | 5342 | $47.50 | $62.50 | 47.50PV |
| Nutmeg 5 ml | 3599 | $13.25 | $17.43 | 13.25PV |
| Orange 15 ml | 3602 | $11.00 | $14.47 | 11PV |
| Oregano 15 ml | 3605 | $28.50 | $37.50 | 28.50PV |
| Palmarosa 15 ml | 3077 | $20.25 | $26.64 | 20.25PV |
| Palo Santo 5 ml | 3607 | $35.50 | $46.71 | 35.50PV |
| Patchouli 15 ml | 3608 | $34.75 | $45.72 | 34.75PV |
| Peppermint 15 ml | 3614 | $22.00 | $28.95 | 22PV |
| Petitgrain 5 ml | 3617 | $35.75 | $47.04 | 35.75PV |
| Pine 15 ml | 3618 | $15.50 | $20.39 | 15.50PV |
| Ravintsara 5 ml | 3620 | $28.50 | $37.50 | 28.50PV |
| Roman Chamomile 5 ml | 3512 | $41.00 | $53.95 | 41PV |
| Rose 5 ml | 3623 | $191.00 | $251.32 | 93.75PV |
| Rosemary 15 ml | 3626 | $16.00 | $21.05 | 16PV |
| Royal Hawaiian Sandalwood 5 ml | 4746 | $97.50 | $128.29 | 97.50PV |
| Sacred Frankincense 5 ml | 3550 | $43.50 | $57.24 | 43.50PV |
| Sacred Frankincense 15 ml | 3552 | $92.50 | $121.71 | 92.50PV |
| Sacred Sandalwood 5 ml | 19651 | $99.75 | $131.25 | 74.75PV |
| Sage 15 ml | 3632 | $29.00 | $38.16 | 29PV |
| Spearmint 5 ml | 3638 | $11.00 | $14.47 | 11PV |
| Tangerine 15 ml | 3644 | $16.50 | $21.71 | 16.50PV |
| Tea Tree 15 ml | 3587 | $26.75 | $35.20 | 26.75PV |
| Thyme 15 ml | 3650 | $34.75 | $45.72 | 34.75PV |
| Tsuga 5 ml | 3352 | $24.75 | $32.57 | 24.75PV |
| Valerian 5 ml | 3648 | $38.50 | $50.66 | 38.50PV |
| Vetiver 5 ml | 3651 | $21.25 | $27.96 | 21.25PV |
| Wintergreen 15 ml | 3658 | $18.25 | $24.01 | 18.25PV |
| Xiang Mao 5 ml | 4658 | $27.50 | $36.18 | 27.50PV |
| Ylang Ylang 15 ml | 3659 | $42.00 | $55.26 | 42PV |

# BLENDS

| Essential Oil Blends | Item | WhSl | Retail | PV |
|---|---|---|---|---|
| 3 Wise Men 15 ml | 3426 | $90.50 | $119.08 | 90.5 |
| Abundance 15 ml | 3300 | $38.00 | $50.00 | 38 |
| Acceptance 5 ml | 3303 | $41.00 | $53.95 | 41 |
| Animal Scents Infect Away 15 ml | 5271 | $25.75 | $33.88 | 19.5 |
| Animal Scents Mendwell 15 ml | 5269 | $18.25 | $24.01 | 13.75 |
| Animal Scents ParaGize 15 ml | 5270 | $11.00 | $14.47 | 8.25 |
| Animal Scents PuriClean 15 ml | 5268 | $24.50 | $32.24 | 18.5 |
| Animal Scents RepelAroma 15 ml | 5272 | $13.00 | $17.11 | 9.75 |
| Animal Scents T-Away 15 ml | 5273 | $16.75 | $22.04 | 12.5 |
| AromaEase 5 ml | 4749 | $35.75 | $47.04 | 35.75 |
| Aroma Life 15 ml | 3306 | $49.25 | $64.80 | 49.25 |
| Aroma Siez 15 ml | 3309 | $32.50 | $42.76 | 32.5 |
| Australian Blue 15 ml | 3311 | $69.25 | $91.12 | 69.25 |
| Awaken 5 ml | 3349 | $21.00 | $27.63 | 21 |
| Believe 15 ml | 4661 | $38.50 | $50.66 | 38.5 |
| Brain Power 5 ml | 3313 | $66.75 | $87.83 | 66.75 |
| Build Your Dream 5 ml | 4834 | $60.50 | $79.61 | 60.5 |
| Christmas Spirit 5 ml | 3356 | $10.50 | $13.82 | 10.5 |
| Citrus Fresh 15 ml | 3318 | $15.75 | $20.72 | 15.75 |
| Clarity 15 ml | 3321 | $41.75 | $54.93 | 41.75 |
| Common Sense 5 ml | 3091 | $35.50 | $46.71 | 33.5 |
| Cool Azul 15 ml | 5399 | $77.00 | $101.32 | 77 |
| DiGize 15 ml | 3324 | $33.75 | $44.41 | 33.75 |
| Dragon Time 15 ml | 3327 | $50.25 | $66.12 | 50.25 |
| Dream Catcher 15 ml | 3330 | $74.25 | $97.70 | 74.25 |
| Egyptian Gold 5 ml | 3332 | $43.25 | $56.91 | 43.25 |
| En-R-Gee 15 ml | 3336 | $25.50 | $33.55 | 25.5 |
| Endoflex 15 ml | 3333 | $28.25 | $37.17 | 28.25 |
| Envision 5 ml | 3337 | $19.25 | $25.33 | 19.25 |
| Exodus II 5 ml | 3338 | $24.00 | $31.58 | 24 |
| Forgiveness 5 ml | 3339 | $54.00 | $71.05 | 54 |
| Fulfill Your Destiny 5 ml | 21284 | $34.75 | $45.72 | 34.75 |
| Gathering 5 ml | 3342 | $30.50 | $40.13 | 30.5 |
| Gentle Baby 5 ml | 3362 | $21.75 | $28.62 | 21.75 |
| GLF 15 ml | 3340 | $135.00 | $177.63 | 135 |
| Gratitude 5 ml | 3346 | $27.00 | $35.53 | 27 |
| Grounding 5 ml | 3348 | $18.25 | $24.01 | 18.25 |
| Harmony 15 ml | 3351 | $71.75 | $94.41 | 71.75 |
| Highest Potential 5 ml | 3373 | $36.50 | $48.03 | 36.5 |
| Hope 5 ml | 3357 | $58.75 | $77.30 | 58.75 |
| Humility 5 ml | 3354 | $27.00 | $35.53 | 27 |
| ImmuPower 15 ml | 3363 | $64.50 | $84.87 | 64.5 |
| Inner Child 5 ml | 3360 | $30.50 | $40.13 | 30.5 |
| Inspiration 15 ml | 3366 | $62.00 | $81.58 | 62 |
| Into The Future 5 ml | 3369 | $27.00 | $35.53 | 27 |
| Joy 15 ml | 3372 | $43.00 | $56.58 | 43 |
| Juva Cleanse 15 ml | 3395 | $109.75 | $144.41 | 109.75 |
| JuvaFlex 5 ml | 3374 | $28.75 | $37.83 | 28.75 |

| Essential Oil Blends (cont) | Item | WhSl | Retail | PV |
|---|---|---|---|---|
| Kidscents GeneYus  5 ml | 5310 | $45.00 | $59.21 | 45 |
| Kidscents Owie        5 ml | 5308 | $31.50 | $41.45 | 31.5 |
| Kidscents Sleepyize 5 ml | 5307 | $17.25 | $22.70 | 17.25 |
| Kidscents SniffleEase 5 ml | 5306 | $18.25 | $24.01 | 18.25 |
| Kidscents TummyGize 5 ml | 5305 | $13.00 | $17.11 | 13 |
| Lady Sclareol 15 ml | 3376 | $56.25 | $74.01 | 56.25 |
| Light The Fire 5 ml | 5304 | $46.00 | $60.53 | 46 |
| Live With Passion 5 ml | 3392 | $75.00 | $98.68 | 75 |
| Live Your Passion 5 ml | 5766 | $57.25 | $75.33 | 57.25 |
| Longevity 15 ml | 3388 | $36.75 | $48.36 | 36.75 |
| M-Grain 15 ml | 3387 | $45.25 | $59.54 | 45.25 |
| Magnify Your Purpose 5 ml | 3377 | $36.50 | $48.03 | 36.5 |
| Melrose 15 ml | 3378 | $20.25 | $26.64 | 20.25 |
| Mister 15 ml | 3381 | $38.75 | $50.99 | 38.75 |
| Motivation 5 ml | 3384 | $52.50 | $69.08 | 52.5 |
| Oola Balance 5 ml | 5022 | $30.50 | $40.13 | 30.5 |
| Oola Faith 5 ml | 5056 | $55.25 | $72.70 | 55.25 |
| Oola Family 5 ml | 5055 | $23.25 | $30.59 | 23.25 |
| Oola Field 5 ml | 5054 | $25.75 | $33.88 | 25.75 |
| Oola Finance 5 ml | 5053 | $33.25 | $43.75 | 33.25 |
| Oola Fitness 5 ml | 5057 | $23.00 | $30.26 | 23 |
| Oola Friends 5 ml | 5052 | $26.50 | $34.87 | 26.5 |
| Oola Fun 5 ml | 5051 | $41.00 | $53.95 | 41 |
| Oola Grow 5 ml | 5021 | $41.00 | $53.95 | 41 |
| Panaway 15 ml | 3390 | $81.75 | $107.57 | 81.75 |
| Panaway 5 ml | 3391 | $36.25 | $47.70 | 36.25 |
| Peace & Calming 5 ml | 3398 | $34.75 | $45.72 | 34.75 |
| Peace & Calming II 5 ml | 5327 | $21.25 | $27.96 | 21.25 |
| Present Time 5 ml | 3396 | $89.00 | $117.11 | 89 |
| Progessence Plus 15ml | 4640 | $38.50 | $50.66 | 38.5 |
| Purification 5 ml | 3389 | $15.75 | $20.72 | 15.75 |
| R.C. 5 ml | 3409 | $10.50 | $13.82 | 10.5 |
| Raven 15 ml | 3402 | $35.75 | $47.04 | 35.75 |
| Release 15 ml | 3408 | $39.25 | $51.64 | 39.25 |
| Relieve It 15 ml | 3411 | $48.00 | $63.16 | 48 |
| Rutavala 5 ml | 3419 | $32.50 | $42.76 | 32.5 |
| Sacred Mountain 15 ml | 3414 | $36.75 | $48.36 | 36.75 |
| Sara 5 ml | 3417 | $26.50 | $34.87 | 26.5 |
| SclarEssence 15 ml | 3418 | $31.50 | $41.45 | 31.5 |
| Sensation 5 ml | 3420 | $34.25 | $45.07 | 34.25 |
| Shutran 15ml | 4835 | $77.25 | $101.64 | 77.25 |
| Slique Essence 15ml | 4586 | $26.75 | $35.20 | 26.75 |
| Stress Away 15 ml | 4630 | $30.50 | $40.13 | 30.5 |
| Surrender 5 ml | 3424 | $26.75 | $35.20 | 26.75 |
| The Gift 5 ml | 6500 | $46.25 | $60.86 | 46.25 |
| Thieves 15 ml | 3423 | $34.75 | $45.72 | 34.75 |
| Transformation 15 ml | 3060 | $70.75 | $93.09 | 70.75 |
| Trauma Life 5 ml | 6350 | $50.50 | $66.45 | 50.5 |
| Valor 5 ml | 3430 | $39.75 | $52.30 | 39.75 |
| White Angelica 5 ml | 3428 | $28.75 | $37.83 | 28.75 |

# VITALITY™ - DIETARY SUPPLEMENTS

| Vitality Dietary Essential Oils | Item | WhSl | Retail | PV |
|---|---|---|---|---|
| Basil Vitality 5 ml | 5583 | $11.00 | $14.47 | 11 |
| Bergamot Vitality 5 ml | 5616 | $13.25 | $17.43 | 13.25 |
| Black Pepper Vitality 5 ml | 5617 | $19.25 | $25.33 | 19.25 |
| Cardamom Vitality 5 ml | 5634 | $26.00 | $34.21 | 26 |
| Carrot Seed Vitality 5 ml | 5618 | $22.25 | $29.28 | 22.25 |
| *Celery Seed Vitality 5 ml | 5584 | $12.00 | $15.79 | 12 |
| Cinnamon Bark Vitality 5 ml | 5585 | $24.75 | $32.57 | 24.75 |
| Citrus Fresh Vitality 5 ml | 5619 | $7.50 | $9.87 | 7.5 |
| Clove Vitality 5 ml | 5620 | $7.50 | $9.87 | 7.5 |
| Copaiba Vitality 5 ml | 5632 | $22.00 | $28.95 | 22 |
| Coriander Vitality 5 ml | 5635 | $32.25 | $42.43 | 32.25 |
| DiGize Vitality 5 ml | 5621 | $14.00 | $18.42 | 14 |
| Dill Vitality 5 ml | 5622 | $16.25 | $21.38 | 16.25 |
| Endoflex Vitality 5 ml | 5623 | $12.75 | $16.78 | 12.75 |
| Fennel Vitality 5 ml | 5636 | $9.00 | $11.84 | 9 |
| Frankincense Vitality 5 ml | 5587 | $30.50 | $40.13 | 30.5 |
| German Chamomile Vitality 5 ml | 5637 | $37.50 | $49.34 | 37.5 |
| Ginger Vitality 5 ml | 5588 | $13.50 | $17.76 | 13.5 |
| GLF Vitality 5 ml | 19168 | $64.00 | $84.21 | 64 |
| Grapefruit Vitality 5 ml | 5624 | $7.75 | $10.20 | 7.75 |
| Jade Lemon Vitality 5 ml | 5589 | $11.00 | $14.47 | 11 |
| Juva Cleanse Vitality 5 ml | 5638 | $52.25 | $68.75 | 52.25 |
| JuvaFlex Vitality 5 ml | 5639 | $28.75 | $37.83 | 28.75 |
| *Laurus Nobilis Vitality 5 ml | 19174 | $25.00 | $32.89 | 25 |
| Lavender Vitality 5 ml | 5590 | $12.00 | $15.79 | 12 |
| Lemon Vitality 5 ml | 5625 | $6.25 | $8.22 | 6.25 |
| Lemongrass Vitality 5 ml | 5626 | $6.25 | $8.22 | 6.25 |
| Lime Vitality 5 ml | 5591 | $5.75 | $7.57 | 5.75 |
| Longevity Vitality 5 ml | 5640 | $15.75 | $20.72 | 15.75 |
| Marjoram Vitality 5 ml | 5592 | $14.75 | $19.41 | 14.75 |
| Mountain Savory Vitality 5 ml | 19171 | $25.50 | $33.55 | 25.5 |
| Nutmeg Vitality 5 ml | 5633 | $13.25 | $17.43 | 13.25 |
| Orange Vitality 5 ml | 5627 | $6.00 | $7.89 | 6 |
| Oregano Vitality 5 ml | 5594 | $12.00 | $15.79 | 12 |
| Peppermint Vitality 5 ml | 5628 | $10.25 | $13.49 | 10.25 |
| Rosemary Vitality 5 ml | 5629 | $7.75 | $10.20 | 7.75 |
| Sage Vitality 5 ml | 5642 | $12.75 | $16.78 | 12.75 |
| SclarEssence Vitality 5 ml | 19175 | $15.00 | $19.74 | 15 |
| Spearmint Vitality 5 ml | 5595 | $11.00 | $14.47 | 11 |
| Tangerine Vitality 5 ml | 5630 | $7.75 | $10.20 | 7.75 |
| *Tarragon Vitality 5 ml | 5643 | $21.00 | $27.63 | 21 |
| Thieves Vitality 5 ml | 5631 | $14.75 | $19.41 | 14.75 |
| Thyme Vitality 5 ml | 5597 | $14.50 | $19.08 | 14.5 |

* Only available through the Vitality™ Line

# ROLL-ONS

| Essential Oil Roll-Ons | Item | WhSl | Retail | PV |
|---|---|---|---|---|
| Breathe Again Roll-On 10 ml | 3528 | $26.50 | $34.87 | 26.5 |
| Deep Relief Roll-On 10 ml | 3534 | $27.50 | $36.18 | 27.5 |
| Rutavala Roll-On 10 ml | 4471 | $36.75 | $48.36 | 36.75 |
| Stress Away Roll-On 10 ml | 4472 | $29.50 | $38.82 | 29.5 |
| Tranquil Roll-On 10 ml | 3533 | $29.50 | $38.82 | 29.5 |
| Valor Roll-On 10 ml | 3529 | $49.75 | $65.46 | 49.75 |

# DIFFUSERS

| Diffusers | Item | WhSl | Retail | PV |
|---|---|---|---|---|
| Aria Ultrasonic Diffuser | 4524 | $231.75 | $304.93 | 139.25 |
| AromaLux Atomizing Diffuser | 4695 | $113.00 | $148.68 | 67.75 |
| AromaLux Atomizing Diffuser (Top) | 4694 | $4.50 | $5.92 | 0 |
| Desert Mist Ultrasonic Diffuser | 21558 | $63.75 | $83.88 | 38.25 |
| Dewdrop Diffuser | 5330 | $63.75 | $83.88 | 38.25 |
| Gentle Mist Personal Diffuser | 5341 | $39.75 | $52.30 | 20 |
| KidScents Dino Land US Diffuser | 5332 | $94.50 | $124.34 | 47.25 |
| KidScents Dino Land (Cover) | 5334 | $43.00 | $56.58 | 0 |
| KidScents Dolphin Reef US Diffuser | 5333 | $97.50 | $128.29 | 48.75 |
| KidScents Dolphin Reef (Cover) | 5335 | $46.00 | $60.53 | 0 |
| Orb Diffuser | 5227 | $26.50 | $34.87 | 16 |
| Orb Diffuser (Replacement Wicks) 3 PK | 5256 | $0.75 | $0.99 | 0 |
| Rainstone Ultrasonic Diffuser | 5331 | $174.75 | $229.93 | 104.75 |
| Resin Burner | 4880 | $33.75 | $44.41 | 16.75 |
| Resin | 4881 | $16.75 | $22.04 | 16.75 |
| Sundance Diffuser | 5490 | $94.50 | $124.34 | 47.25 |
| Sundance Diffuser (Cover) | 5491 | $43.00 | $56.58 | 0 |
| USB Diffuser (Black) | 5223 | $23.25 | $30.59 | 12.25 |
| USB Diffuser (Purple) | 5226 | $23.25 | $30.59 | 12.25 |

# MASSAGE OILS

| Massage Oils | Size | Item | WhSl | Retail | PV |
|---|---|---|---|---|---|
| Cel-Lite Magic Massage Oil | 8 fl. oz. | 3035 | $32.75 | $43.09 | 32.75 |
| Dragon Time Massage Oil | 8 fl. oz. | 3034 | $35.75 | $47.04 | 35.75 |
| Ortho Ease Massage Oil | 8 fl. oz. | 3033 | $35.75 | $47.04 | 35.75 |
| Ortho Sport Massage Oil | 8 fl. oz. | 3032 | $35.75 | $47.04 | 35.75 |
| Relaxation Massage Oil | 8 fl. oz. | 3037 | $35.75 | $47.04 | 35.75 |
| Sensation Massage Oil | 8 fl. oz. | 3036 | $35.75 | $47.04 | 35.75 |
| V-6 Vegetable Oil Complex | 8 fl. oz. | 3031 | $22.25 | $29.28 | 22.25 |
| V-6 Vegetable Oil Complex | 32 fl. oz. | 3030 | $50.00 | $65.79 | 50 |

# COLLECTIONS

| Essential Oil Collections | Item | WhSl | Retail | PV |
|---|---|---|---|---|
| Active & Fit Kit | 5502 | $87.50 | $115.13 | 77.25 |
| Essence of the Season | 3118 | $82.00 | $107.89 | 82 |
| Everyday Oils | 3695 | $138.75 | $182.57 | 138.75 |
| Feelings | 3125 | $181.00 | $238.16 | 181 |
| Golden Touch I | 3130 | $92.25 | $121.38 | 92.25 |
| Infused 7 Kit | 5058 | $205.75 | $270.72 | 205.75 |
| Oils of Ancient Scripture | 19341 | $205.75 | $270.72 | 205.75 |
| Premier Aroma Collection | 3100 | $2,162.00 | $2,844.74 | 2162 |
| Raindrop Technique | 3137 | $138.75 | $182.57 | 138.75 |
| Reconnect Collection | 5340 | $205.75 | $270.72 | 205.75 |
| Select 30 Oil Collection | 5763 | $386.25 | $508.22 | 386.25 |

# THIEVES® LINE

| Thieves | Size | Item | WhSl | Retail | PV |
|---|---|---|---|---|---|
| Thieves | 15 ml | 3423 | $34.75 | $45.72 | 34.75 |
| Thieves AromaBright Toothpaste (4oz) | 1 Ct | 3039 | $10.50 | $13.82 | 10.5 |
| Thieves AromaBright Toothpaste (2oz) | 5 pk | 5351 | $28.75 | $37.83 | 28.75 |
| Thieves Automatic Dishwasher Powder | 16 oz | 5762 | $25.50 | $33.55 | 25.5 |
| Thieves Cleansing Soap | 3.45 oz | 3679 | $10.50 | $13.82 | 10.5 |
| Thieves Cough Drops | 30 ct | 5760 | $20.50 | $26.97 | 20.5 |
| Thieves Dental Floss | 1 ct | 4463122 | $3.25 | $4.28 | 3.25 |
| Thieves Dental Floss | 3 pk | 4464122 | $9.00 | $11.84 | 9 |
| Thieves Dentarome Plus Toothpaste | 4 oz | 3738 | $6.75 | $8.88 | 6.75 |
| Thieves Dentarome Ultra Toothpaste | 4 oz | 20194 | $9.00 | $11.84 | 9 |
| Thieves Dish Soap | 12 fl. oz | 5350 | $14.00 | $18.42 | 14 |
| Thieves Foaming Hand Soap (8 fl. oz) | 1 ct | 3674 | $13.25 | $17.43 | 13.25 |
| Thieves Foaming Hand Soap (8 fl. oz) | 3 pk | 3643 | $36.50 | $48.03 | 36.5 |
| Thieves Foaming Hand Soap Refill | 32 fl. oz | 3594 | $39.50 | $51.97 | 39.5 |
| Thieves Fresh Essence Plus Mouthwash | 8 fl. oz | 3683 | $11.25 | $14.80 | 11.25 |
| Thieves Fruit & Veggie Soak | 16 fl. oz | 5352 | $19.75 | $25.99 | 19.75 |
| Thieves Fruit & Veggie Spray | 2 fl. oz | 5348 | $8.50 | $11.18 | 8.5 |
| Thieves Hard Lozenges | 30 ct | 3282 | $19.00 | $25.00 | 19 |
| Thieves Home Cleaning Kit | | 20421 | $79.75 | $104.93 | 62.5 |
| Thieves Household Cleaner | 14.4fl. oz | 3743 | $22.50 | $29.61 | 22.5 |
| Thieves Household Cleaner Refill | 64 fl. oz | 4475 | $87.75 | $115.46 | 87.75 |
| Thieves Laundry Soap | 32 fl oz | 5349 | $29.50 | $38.82 | 29.5 |
| Thieves Mints | 30 ct | 5138 | $13.00 | $17.11 | 13 |
| Thieves Mints | 3 pk | 5140 | $35.50 | $46.71 | 35.5 |
| Thieves Spray | 1 fl oz | 3265 | $9.25 | $12.17 | 9.25 |
| Thieves Spray | 3 pk | 3266 | $24.50 | $32.24 | 24.5 |
| Thieves Vitality | 5 ml | 5631 | $14.75 | $19.41 | 14.75 |
| Thieves Waterless Hand Purifier | 1 fl oz | 3621 | $5.00 | $6.58 | 5 |
| Thieves Waterless Hand Purifier 3 pk | 1 fl. oz | 3622 | $14.00 | $18.42 | 14 |
| Thieves Waterless Hand Purifier | 7.6 fl oz | 5142 | $27.25 | $35.86 | 27.25 |
| Thieves Wipes | 30 ct | 3756 | $13.50 | $17.76 | 13.5 |

# SUPPLEMENTS

| Foundation Nutrition | Size | Item | WhSl | Retail | PV |
|---|---|---|---|---|---|
| Balance Complete | 26.4 oz | 3292 | $51.25 | $67.43 | 51.25 |
| Core Supplements | | 3506 | $184.00 | $242.11 | 184 |
| Inner Defense | 30 ct | 3295 | $27.50 | $36.18 | 27.5 |
| Life 9 | 30 ct | 18299 | $29.50 | $38.82 | 29.5 |
| Longevity Softgels | 30 ct | 3289 | $32.75 | $43.09 | 32.75 |
| Master Formula | 30 ct | 5292 | $82.00 | $107.89 | 82 |
| Mineral Essence | 3.6 fl oz | 3222 | $29.50 | $38.82 | 29.5 |
| OmegaGize | 120 ct | 3097 | $60.50 | $79.61 | 60.5 |
| Super B | 60 ct | 3240 | $20.25 | $26.64 | 20.25 |
| Super C (Tablet) | 120 ct | 3242 | $29.50 | $38.82 | 29.5 |
| Super C (Chewable) | 90 ct | 3251 | $32.75 | $43.09 | 32.75 |

| Cleansing Nutrition | Size | Item | WhSl | Retail | PV |
|---|---|---|---|---|---|
| 5 Day Nutritive Cleanse | | 4890 | $124.75 | $164.14 | 124.75 |
| Cleansing Trio | | 3115 | $90.25 | $118.75 | 90.25 |
| ComforTone | 150 ct | 3204 | $34.75 | $45.72 | 34.75 |
| Digest & Cleanse | 30 ct | 3293 | $30.50 | $40.13 | 30.5 |
| ICP | 8 oz | 3208 | $26.50 | $34.87 | 26.5 |
| JuvaPower | 8 oz | 3276 | $44.00 | $57.89 | 44 |
| JuvaTone | 150 ct | 3214 | $36.75 | $48.36 | 36.75 |
| MultiGreens | 120 ct | 3248 | $41.00 | $53.95 | 41 |
| ParaFree | 180 ct | 6201 | $92.50 | $121.71 | 92.5 |
| Rehemogen | 1.8 fl oz | 3264 | $29.50 | $38.82 | 29.5 |

| Targeted Nutrition | Size | Item | WhSl | Retail | PV |
|---|---|---|---|---|---|
| AgliEase | 60 ct | 5764 | $47.00 | $61.84 | 47 |
| AlkaLime | 8 oz | 3199 | $35.75 | $47.04 | 35.75 |
| AlkaLime Stick Packs | 30 ct | 3055 | $29.75 | $39.14 | 29.75 |
| Allerzyme | 90 ct | 3288 | $35.75 | $47.04 | 35.75 |
| AminoWise | 7.32 oz | 20083 | $33.75 | $44.41 | 33.75 |
| BLM | 90 ct | 3234 | $44.00 | $57.89 | 44 |
| CortiStop | 60 ct | 3275 | $56.25 | $74.01 | 56.25 |
| Detoxzyme | 180 ct | 3203 | $43.00 | $56.58 | 43 |
| EndoGize | 60 ct | 3090 | $44.00 | $57.89 | 44 |
| Essentialzymes | 90 ct | 3272 | $41.00 | $53.95 | 41 |
| Essentialzymes-4 | 120 ct | 4645 | $51.25 | $67.43 | 51.25 |
| Femigen | 60 ct | 3206 | $23.25 | $30.59 | 23.25 |
| ImmuPro | 30 ct | 3213 | $34.75 | $45.72 | 34.75 |
| K & B | 1.8 fl oz | 3262 | $30.50 | $40.13 | 30.5 |
| MegaCal | 15.6 oz | 3280 | $41.00 | $53.95 | 41 |
| MindWise | 15 fl oz | 21244 | $61.50 | $80.92 | 61.5 |
| MindWise Single Packets | 30 ct | 20223 | $67.75 | $89.14 | 67.75 |
| PD 80/20 | 30 ct | 3263 | $64.50 | $84.87 | 64.5 |
| Powergize | 60 ct | 4748 | $30.50 | $40.13 | 30.5 |
| Prostate Health | 60 ct | 21016 | $35.75 | $47.04 | 35.75 |
| Pure Protein Complete Chocolate | 29.4 oz | 3298 | $67.00 | $88.16 | 53.75 |
| Pure Protein Complete Vanilla Spice | 26.2 oz | 3301 | $67.00 | $88.16 | 53.75 |
| SleepEssence | 30 ct | 4760 | $25.50 | $33.55 | 25.5 |
| Sulfurzyme (Capsules) | 300 ct | 3243 | $59.25 | $77.96 | 59.25 |
| Sulfurzyme (Powder) | 8 oz | 3241 | $47.25 | $62.17 | 47.25 |
| Super Cal Plus | 60 ct | 20240 | $26.50 | $34.87 | 26.5 |
| Thyromin | 60 ct | 3246 | $43.00 | $56.58 | 43 |

# NINGXIA RED® LINE

| NingXia Red | Size | Item | WhSl | Retail | PV |
|---|---|---|---|---|---|
| NingXia Dried Wolfberries | 16 oz | 6360 | $25.50 | $33.55 | 20.5 |
| NingXia Nitro | 14 ct | 3064 | $39.75 | $52.30 | 39.75 |
| NingXia Red | 2 pk | 3042 | $73.00 | $96.05 | 73 |
| NingXia Red | 4 pk | 3044 | $130.75 | $172.04 | 130.75 |
| NingXia Red | 6 pk | 3045 | $192.75 | $253.62 | 192.75 |
| NingXia Red | 8 pk | 3046 | $250.75 | $329.93 | 250.75 |
| NR Combo Pack | 30ct /2b | 4710 | $152.00 | $200.00 | 152 |
| NingXia Red Singles | 30 ct | 3525 | $87.00 | $114.47 | 87 |
| NingXia Red Singles | 60 ct | 3526 | $169.50 | $223.03 | 169.5 |
| NingXia Red Singles | 90 ct | 3523 | $252.25 | $331.91 | 252.25 |
| NingXia Zyng | 12 ct | 3071 | $35.75 | $47.04 | 26.75 |

# SLIQUE®

| Slique | Size | Item | WhSl | Retail | PV |
|---|---|---|---|---|---|
| Slique Advanced Collection | | 20028 | $185.00 | $243.42 | 159.75 |
| Slique Assist Collection | | 20027 | $105.75 | $139.14 | 105.75 |
| Slique Complete Collection | | 20026 | $352.25 | $463.49 | 309 |
| Slique Maintain Collection | | 20053 | $65.75 | $86.51 | 65.75 |
| Slique Bars | 6 ct | 5024 | $18.25 | $24.01 | 9.25 |
| Slique Bars Chocolate-Coated | 6 ct | 5297 | $18.25 | $24.01 | 9.25 |
| Slique Citraslim | 15 ct | 3056 | $46.25 | $60.86 | 46.25 |
| Slique Essence | 15ml | 4586 | $26.75 | $35.20 | 26.75 |
| Slique Gum | 8 ct | 4579 | $8.00 | $10.53 | 8 |
| Slique Gum 8ct | 3 pk | 4627 | $23.50 | $30.92 | 23.5 |
| Slique Gum 8ct | 12 pk | 4628 | $91.50 | $120.39 | 91.5 |
| Slique Shake | 15 ct | 5552 | $51.25 | $67.43 | 41.25 |
| Slique Tea | 25 ct | 4560 | $20.25 | $26.64 | 20.25 |

# SAVVY MINERALS™

| Savvy Minerals Additional Items | Type | Item | WhSl | Retail | PV |
|---|---|---|---|---|---|
| Brush Set | Brushes | 21257 | $85.00 | $111.84 | 85 |
| Brushes: Bronzer Brush | Brush | 20839 | $28.00 | $36.84 | 28 |
| Brushes: Contour Brush | Brush | 20843 | $34.00 | $44.74 | 34 |
| Brushes: Concealer Brush | Brush | 20844 | $24.00 | $31.58 | 24 |
| Brushes: Eyebrow Brush | Brush | 20845 | $15.00 | $19.74 | 15 |
| Brushes: Eyeliner Brush | Brush | 20846 | $24.00 | $31.58 | 24 |
| Misting Spray | Spray | 21397 | $15.00 | $19.74 | 15 |
| Holiday Collection | | 21952 | $140.00 | $182.21 | 125 |
| Poppy Seed Lip Scrub 23749  Scrub | | 23749 | $28.00 | $36.84 | 28 |

# MAKEUP - SAVVY MINERALS™

| Savvy Minerals | Color | Item | WhSl | Retail | PV |
|---|---|---|---|---|---|
| Blush: Awestruck | Shimmer Soft Pink | 22845 | $27.75 | $36.51 | 27.75 |
| Blush: Captivate | Matte Beige Pink | 22848 | $27.75 | $36.51 | 27.75 |
| Blush: Charisma | Matte Bright Pink | 22852 | $27.75 | $36.51 | 27.75 |
| Blush: I Do Believe You're Blushing | Shimmer Light Plum | 20795 | $27.75 | $36.51 | 27.75 |
| Blush: Passionate | Matte Medium Plum | 20797 | $27.75 | $36.51 | 27.75 |
| Blush: Serene | Matte Soft Coral Peach | 22856 | $27.75 | $36.51 | 27.75 |
| Blush: Smashing | Shimmer Light Peach | 20796 | $27.75 | $36.51 | 27.75 |
| Bronzer: Crowned All Over | Shimmer Light Tan | 20787 | $27.75 | $36.51 | 27.75 |
| Bronzer: Summer Loved | Shimmer Medium Tan | 20788 | $27.75 | $36.51 | 27.75 |
| Foundation: Cool No 1 | Matte Pink Light | 20776 | $44.00 | $57.89 | 44 |
| Foundation: Cool No 2 | Matte Pink Medium | 20775 | $44.00 | $57.89 | 44 |
| Foundation: Cool No 3 | Matte Pink Medum Dark | 20773 | $44.00 | $57.89 | 44 |
| Foundation: Dark No 1 | Matte Tan | 20858 | $44.00 | $57.89 | 44 |
| Foundation: Dark No 2 | Matte Medium Tan | 20859 | $44.00 | $57.89 | 44 |
| Foundation: Dark No 3 | Matte Brown | 20860 | $44.00 | $57.89 | 44 |
| Foundation: Dark No 4 | Matte Dark Brown | 20861 | $44.00 | $57.89 | 44 |
| Foundation: Warm No 1 | Matte Yellow Light | 20777 | $44.00 | $57.89 | 44 |
| Foundation: Warm No 2 | Matte Yellow Medum | 20774 | $44.00 | $57.89 | 44 |
| Foundation: Warm No 3 | Matte Yellow Med Dark | 20772 | $44.00 | $57.89 | 44 |
| Veil: Diamond Dust | Shimmer White | 20793 | $45.00 | $59.21 | 45 |
| Eyeliner: Jet Setter | Black | 20791 | $15.75 | $20.72 | 15.75 |
| Eyeliner: Multitasker | Dark Brown | 20794 | $20.75 | $27.30 | 20.75 |
| Eyeshadow: Best Kept Secret | Matte Nude | 20782 | $15.25 | $20.07 | 15.25 |
| Eyeshadow: Crushin' | Shimmer Nude Peach | 20896 | $15.25 | $20.07 | 15.25 |
| Eyeshadow: Determined | Shimmer Medium Brown | 20781 | $15.25 | $20.07 | 15.25 |
| Eyeshadow: Diffused | Matte Medium Plum | 20894 | $15.25 | $20.07 | 15.25 |
| Eyeshadow: Envy | Shimmer Violet-Gray | 22857 | $15.25 | $20.07 | 15.25 |
| Eyeshadow: Freedom | Shimmer Golden Green | 20856 | $15.25 | $20.07 | 15.25 |
| Eyeshadow: Inspired | Shimmer Light Mauve | 21022 | $15.25 | $20.07 | 15.25 |
| Eyeshadow: Overboard | Shimmer Plum | 22859 | $15.25 | $20.07 | 15.25 |
| Eyeshadow: Residual | Shimmer Pale Beige | 20785 | $15.25 | $20.07 | 15.25 |
| Eyeshadow: Spoiled | Matte Pink | 20784 | $15.25 | $20.07 | 15.25 |
| Eyeshadow: Unscripted | Matte Dark Plum | 20895 | $15.25 | $20.07 | 15.25 |
| Eyeshadow: Wanderlust | Shimmer Pale White | 20783 | $15.25 | $20.07 | 15.25 |
| Lip Gloss: Abundant | Sheer Light Plum | 20825 | $27.50 | $36.18 | 27.5 |
| Lip Gloss: Anchors Aweigh | Medium Dark Mauve | 22072 | $27.50 | $36.18 | 27.5 |
| Lip Gloss: Embrace | Nude Pink | 20832 | $27.50 | $36.18 | 27.5 |
| Lip Gloss: Headliner | Bright Pink | 22073 | $27.50 | $36.18 | 27.5 |
| Lip Gloss: Journey | Bronze Nude | 21689 | $27.50 | $36.18 | 27.5 |
| Lip Gloss: Maven | Medium Dark Mauve | 21688 | $27.50 | $36.18 | 27.5 |
| Lip Stick: Adore | Neutral Pink | 21295 | $22.75 | $29.93 | 22.75 |
| Lip Stick: Bedazzled (Tangerine) | Plum Berry | 21751 | $29.75 | $39.14 | 29.75 |
| Lip Stick: Day Dream | Pale Peachy Nude | 21292 | $22.75 | $29.93 | 22.75 |
| Lip Stick: I Dare You (Tangerine) | Coral Orange | 23021 | $29.75 | $39.14 | 29.75 |
| Lip Stick: It Girl (Tangerine) | Pale Pink Beige | 23020 | $29.75 | $39.14 | 29.75 |
| Lip Stick: Mic Drop (Tangerine) | Bright Pink | 23019 | $29.75 | $39.14 | 29.75 |
| Lip Stick: Miss Congeniality (Tangerine) | Soft Pink | 23022 | $29.75 | $39.14 | 29.75 |
| Lip Stick: On A Whim | Beige Nude | 21293 | $22.75 | $29.93 | 22.75 |
| Lip Stick: Sweet Life (Tangerine) | Bright Fuchsia | 21752 | $29.75 | $39.14 | 29.75 |
| Lip Stick: Uptown Girl | Dusty Rose | 21296 | $22.75 | $29.93 | 22.75 |
| Lip Stick: Wish | Nude Rose | 21294 | $22.75 | $29.93 | 22.75 |

# FACIAL – ART LINE

| ART | Size | Item | WhSl | Retail | PV |
|---|---|---|---|---|---|
| ART Creme Masque | 1 fl oz | 5173 | $48.00 | $63.16 | 48 |
| ART Gentle Cleanser | 3.38 fl oz | 5361 | $33.75 | $44.41 | 33.75 |
| ART Intensive Moisturizer | 1.7 fl oz | 5663 | $67.00 | $88.16 | 67 |
| ART Beauty Masque | 4 pk | 20210 | $47.50 | $62.50 | 47.5 |
| ART Light Moisturizer | 30ml | 5362 | $60.25 | $79.28 | 60.25 |
| ART Refreshing Toner | 4 fl oz | 5360 | $24.75 | $32.57 | 24.75 |
| ART Renewal Serum | 20ml | 5175 | $77.00 | $101.32 | 77 |
| ART Sheerlume Brightening Cream | 30ml | 4833 | $69.75 | $91.78 | 69.75 |
| ART Skin Care System | | 5363 | $113.00 | $148.68 | 113 |

# FACIAL & BODY

| Facial Care | Size | Item | WhSl | Retail | PV |
|---|---|---|---|---|---|
| Boswellia Wrinkle Cream | 2 oz | 5141 | $67.25 | $88.49 | 67.25 |
| Coconut-Lime Body Butter | 2.82 oz | 20225 | $32.25 | $42.43 | 32.25 |
| Essential Beauty Serum | 15 ml | 3782 | $20.75 | $27.30 | 20.75 |
| Genesis Hand & Body Lotion | 8 oz | 3706 | $21.00 | $27.63 | 21 |
| Lavender Hand & Body Lotion | 8 oz | 5201 | $21.25 | $27.96 | 21.25 |
| Lip Balm Cinnamint | 0.16 oz | 5150 | $4.25 | $5.59 | 4.25 |
| Lip Balm Grapefruit | 0.16 oz | 5178 | $4.25 | $5.59 | 4.25 |
| Lip Balm Lavender | 0.16 oz | 5203 | $4.00 | $5.26 | 4 |
| Orange Blossom Facial Wash | 4 fl oz | 5136 | $41.00 | $53.95 | 41 |
| Regenolone Moisturizing Cream | 4 oz | 3729 | $54.50 | $71.71 | 54.5 |
| Rose Ointment | 1 oz | 3709 | $24.50 | $32.24 | 24.5 |
| Satin Facial Scrub, Mint | 2 fl oz | 3735 | $16.75 | $22.04 | 16.75 |
| Sensation Hand & Body Lotion | 8.6 oz | 3707 | $26.50 | $34.87 | 26.5 |
| Wolfberry Eye Cream | 0.5 oz | 5145 | $47.50 | $62.50 | 47.5 |

# SOAP & BODY WASH

| Soaps & Body Gel Size | Size | Item | WhSl | Retail | PV |
|---|---|---|---|---|---|
| Bath & Shower Gel Base | 8 fl oz | 3751 | $16.00 | $21.05 | 16 |
| Dragon Time Bath & Shower Gel | 8 fl oz | 3739 | $20.75 | $27.30 | 20.75 |
| Evening Peace Bath & Shower Gel | 8 fl oz | 3742 | $28.75 | $37.83 | 28.75 |
| Lavender Bath & Shower Gel | 8 fl oz | 5202 | $19.00 | $25.00 | 19 |
| Lavender Foaming Hand Soap | 8 fl oz | 4430 | $11.75 | $15.46 | 11.75 |
| Lavender Foaming Hand Soap | 3 pk | 4431 | $32.25 | $42.43 | 32.25 |
| Lavender Oatmeal Bar Soap | 3.5 oz | 4904 | $10.50 | $13.82 | 10.5 |
| Lemon-Sandalwood Cleansing Soap | 3.5 oz | 3675 | $10.50 | $13.82 | 10.5 |
| Morning Start Bath & Shower Gel | 8 fl oz | 3745 | $19.25 | $25.33 | 19.25 |
| Morning Start Moisturizing Soap | 3.5 oz | 3676 | $10.50 | $13.82 | 10.5 |
| Peppermint-Cedarwood Moisturizing Soap | 3.5 oz | 3677 | $10.50 | $13.82 | 10.5 |
| Sacred Mountain Moisturizing Soap | 3.5 oz | 3671 | $10.50 | $13.82 | 10.5 |
| Sensation Bath & Shower Gel | 8 fl oz | 3748 | $21.25 | $27.96 | 21.25 |
| Thieves Cleansing Soap | 3.5 oz | 3679 | $10.50 | $13.82 | 10.5 |
| Thieves Foaming Hand Soap | 8 fl oz | 3674 | $13.25 | $17.43 | 13.25 |
| Thieves Foaming Hand Soap (8 fl oz) | 3 pk | 3643 | $36.50 | $48.03 | 36.5 |
| Thieves Foaming Hand Soap Refill | 32 fl oz | 3594 | $39.50 | $51.97 | 39.5 |
| Valor Moisturizing Soap | 3.5 oz | 3680 | $12.50 | $16.45 | 12.5 |

# BODY

| Body Care | Size | Item | WhSl | Retail | PV |
|---|---|---|---|---|---|
| Aromaguard Meadow Mist Deodorant | 1.5 oz | 3752 | $11.25 | $14.80 | 11.25 |
| Aromaguard Mountain Mint Deodorant | 1.5 oz | 3753 | $11.25 | $14.80 | 11.25 |
| Bon Voyage Kit | | 4699 | $56.50 | $74.34 | 51.25 |
| Claraderm | 2 fl oz | 3750 | $66.25 | $87.17 | 66.25 |
| Cool Azul Pain Relief Cream | 3.4 fl oz | 5759 | $44.00 | $57.89 | 44 |
| Cool Azul Sports Gel | 3.4 fl oz | 5436 | $41.00 | $53.95 | 41 |
| Insect Repellent | 6 fl oz | 20701 | $38.75 | $50.99 | 38.75 |
| Lavaderm After-Sun Spray | 2 fl oz | 20673 | $24.75 | $32.57 | 24.75 |
| Lavaderm Cooling Mist | 2 fl oz | 3249 | $14.00 | $18.42 | 14 |
| Lavender Calming Bath Bombs | 4 ct | 20671 | $25.75 | $33.88 | 25.75 |
| Mineral Sunscreen Lotion | 3 oz | 20667 | $26.75 | $35.20 | 26.75 |
| Mirah Shave Oil | 2 fl oz | 5156 | $23.25 | $30.59 | 23.25 |
| Prenolone Plus Body Cream | 1.94 oz | 3732 | $37.75 | $49.67 | 37.75 |
| Progessence Plus | 15ml | 4640 | $38.50 | $50.66 | 38.5 |
| Protec | 8 fl oz | 3231 | $86.75 | $114.14 | 86.75 |
| Stress Away Relaxing Bath Bombs | 4 ct | 20674 | $25.75 | $33.88 | 25.75 |

# HAIR

| Hair CareSize | Size | Item | WhSl | Retail | PV |
|---|---|---|---|---|---|
| Copaiba Vanilla Moisturizing Shampoo | 10 fl oz | 5194121 | $23.25 | $30.59 | 23.25 |
| Copaiba Vanilla Moisturizing Conditioner | 10 fl oz | 5195121 | $23.25 | $30.59 | 23.25 |
| Lavender Mint Daily Shampoo | 10 fl oz | 5191121 | $20.25 | $26.64 | 20.25 |
| Lavender Mint Daily Conditioner | 10 fl oz | 5192121 | $20.25 | $26.64 | 20.25 |
| Lavender Shampoo | 8 fl oz | 5100 | $20.25 | $26.64 | 20.25 |
| Lavender Conditioner | 8 fl oz | 5102 | $20.25 | $26.64 | 20.25 |

# DENTAL

| Dental Care | Size | Item | WhSl | Retail | PV |
|---|---|---|---|---|---|
| Kidscents Toothpaste | 4 oz | 4574 | $7.50 | $9.87 | 7.5 |
| Thieves Aromabright Toothpaste | 4 oz | 3039 | $10.50 | $13.82 | 10.5 |
| Thieves Aromabright Toothpaste | 5- 2 oz tubes | 5351 | $28.75 | $37.83 | 28.75 |
| Thieves Dentarome Plus Toothpaste | 4 oz | 3738 | $6.75 | $8.88 | 6.75 |
| Thieves Dentarome Ultra Toothpaste | 4 oz | 20194 | $9.00 | $11.84 | 9 |
| Thieves Fresh Essence Plus Mouthwash | 8 fl oz | 3683 | $11.25 | $14.80 | 11.25 |
| Thieves Dental Floss | 1 ct | 4463122 | $3.25 | $4.28 | 3.25 |
| Thieves Dental Floss | 3 pk | 4464122 | $9.00 | $11.84 | 9 |

# MEN'S

| Men's Care | Size | Item | WhSl | Retail | PV |
|---|---|---|---|---|---|
| Shutran | 15ml | 4835 | $77.25 | $101.64 | 77.25 |
| Shutran 3-in-1 Men's Wash | 8 fl oz | 20483 | $32.00 | $42.11 | 32 |
| Shutran 3-in-1 Men's Wash | 3 fl oz | 20631 | $16.00 | $21.05 | 16 |
| Shutran Aftershave Lotion | 1.76 oz | 5710 | $26.75 | $35.20 | 26.75 |
| Shutran Bar Soap | 6 oz | 5711 | $20.25 | $26.64 | 20.25 |
| Shutran Beard Oil | 1 fl oz | 19802 | $15.00 | $19.74 | 15 |
| Shutran Shave Cream | 2.5 oz | 5157 | $20.25 | $26.64 | 20.25 |

# SEEDLINGS™

| Seedlings | Size | Item | WhSl | Retail | PV |
|---|---|---|---|---|---|
| Seedlings Baby Lotion, Calm | 4 oz | 20438 | $19.75 | $25.99 | 19.75 |
| Seedlings Baby Oil, Calm | 2.5 fl oz | 20373 | $24.25 | $31.91 | 24.25 |
| Seedlings Baby Wash & Shampoo, Calm | 8 fl oz | 20404 | $20.75 | $27.30 | 20.75 |
| Seedlings Baby Wipes, Calm | 72 ct | 20428 | $11.75 | $15.46 | 11.75 |
| Seedlings Diaper Rash Cream | 2 oz | 20398 | $27.75 | $36.51 | 27.75 |
| Seedlings Linen Spray, Calm | 2.7 fl oz | 20384 | $16.75 | $22.04 | 16.75 |

# KIDSCENTS®

| Kidscents | Size | Item | WhSl | Retail | PV |
|---|---|---|---|---|---|
| KidScents Bath Gel | 8 fl oz | 3684 | $16.25 | $21.38 | 16.25 |
| KidScents Dino Land Ultrasonic Diffuser | | 5332 | $94.50 | $124.34 | 47.25 |
| KidScents Dino Land (Cover) | | 5334 | $43.00 | $56.58 | 0 |
| KidScents Dolphin Reef Ultrasonic Diffuser | | 5333 | $97.50 | $128.29 | 48.75 |
| KidScents Dolphin Reef (Cover) | | 5335 | $46.00 | $60.53 | 0 |
| KidScents GeneYus | 5 ml | 5310 | $45.00 | $59.21 | 45 |
| KidScents Lotion | 7.76 fl oz | 3682 | $22.25 | $29.28 | 22.25 |
| KidScents MightyVites | 120 ct | 20557 | $39.75 | $52.30 | 39.75 |
| KidScents MightyZyme | 90 ct | 3259 | $39.75 | $52.30 | 39.75 |
| KidScents Owie | 5 ml | 5308 | $31.50 | $41.45 | 31.5 |
| KidScents Shampoo | 7.25 fl oz | 3686 | $16.50 | $21.71 | 16.5 |
| KidScents Sleepylze | 5 ml | 5307 | $17.25 | $22.70 | 17.25 |
| KidScents SniffleEase | 5 ml | 5306 | $18.25 | $24.01 | 18.25 |
| KidScents Tender Tush | 1.8 oz | 3689 | $27.75 | $36.51 | 27.75 |
| KidScents Toothpaste | 4 oz | 4574 | $7.50 | $9.87 | 7.5 |
| KidScents TummyGize | 5 ml | 5305 | $13.00 | $17.11 | 13 |

# ANIMAL SCENTS®

| Animal Scents | Size | Item | WhSl | Retail | PV |
|---|---|---|---|---|---|
| Animal Scents Cat Treats | 4 oz | 21399 | $8.75 | $11.51 | 8.75 |
| Animal Scents Dental Pet Chews | 10 ct | 5761 | $20.25 | $26.64 | 20.25 |
| Animal Scents Infect Away | 15 ml | 5271 | $25.75 | $33.88 | 19.5 |
| Animal Scents Mendwell | 15 ml | 5269 | $18.25 | $24.01 | 13.75 |
| Animal Scents Ointment | 6.3 oz | 5165 | $24.75 | $32.57 | 12.25 |
| Animal Scents ParaGize | 15 ml | 5270 | $11.00 | $14.47 | 8.25 |
| Animal Scents PuriClean | 15 ml | 5268 | $24.50 | $32.24 | 18.5 |
| Animal Scents RepelAroma | 15 ml | 5272 | $13.00 | $17.11 | 9.75 |
| Animal Scents Shampoo | 8 fl oz | 5167 | $16.25 | $21.38 | 8 |
| Animal Scents T-Away | 15 ml | 5273 | $16.75 | $22.04 | 12.5 |

# COOKWARE

| Titanium Cookware | Size | Item | WhSl | Retail | PV |
|---|---|---|---|---|---|
| Frying Pan | 20x5 cm | 4060 | $151.50 | $199.34 | 75.75 |
| Frying Pan | 28x5 cm | 4061 | $205.50 | $270.39 | 102.75 |
| High-Rim Frying Pan | 20x7 cm | 4056 | $205.50 | $270.39 | 102.75 |
| High-Rim Frying Pan | 28x7 cm | 4064 | $227.00 | $298.68 | 113.5 |
| Sauce Pan | 20x13 cm | 4057 | $227.00 | $298.68 | 113.5 |
| Glass Lid | 20 cm | 4058 | $20.50 | $26.97 | 10.25 |
| Glass Lid | 28 cm | 4065 | $26.00 | $34.21 | 13 |
| Steamer | 20 cm | 4059 | $64.75 | $85.20 | 32.38 |

# HEALTHY EATING & COOKING

| Healthy Cooking | Size | Item | WhSl | Retail | PV |
|---|---|---|---|---|---|
| Gary's True Grit Einkorn Flour | 32 oz | 5043 | $8.50 | $11.18 | 4.25 |
| Gary's True Grit Pancake and Waffle Mix | 32 oz | 5300 | $8.50 | $11.18 | 4.25 |
| Gary's True Grit Gluten Free Pancake & Waffle Mix | 16 oz | 5298 | $6.50 | $8.55 | 3.25 |
| Gary's True Grit Granola | 12 oz | 5751 | $7.00 | $9.21 | 3.5 |
| Gary's True Grit Granola | 3 pk | 19501 | $20.50 | $26.97 | 10.25 |
| Gary's TG Chocolate Coated Wolfberry Crisp Bars | 10 ct | 5758 | $17.25 | $22.70 | 9.25 |
| GTG Einkorn Rotini Pasta | 17.6 oz | 5750 | $8.50 | $11.18 | 4.25 |
| GTG Einkorn Spaghetti | 8 oz | 5301 | $4.50 | $5.92 | 2.25 |
| GTG NingXia Berry Syrup | 8 fl oz | 19080 | $9.75 | $12.83 | 9.75 |
| Yacon Syrup | 8 fl oz | 4570 | $37.75 | $49.67 | 18.75 |

# ACCESSORIES, SAMPLES, & DIY

| Nutritional Accessories | Item | WhSl | Retail | PV |
|---|---|---|---|---|
| Blender Bottle (Green) | 4609 | $6.00 | $7.89 | 0 |
| Blender Bottle (Purple) | 4622 | $6.00 | $7.89 | 0 |
| Core Vitality Case (Purple) | 5160 | $14.25 | $18.75 | 0 |
| Core Vitality Case (Teal) | 5660 | $14.25 | $18.75 | 0 |
| From Our Fields To Your Table Cookbook | 5689 | $16.75 | $22.04 | 0 |
| HydroGize Water Bottle - Purple (15 fl oz capacity) | 5775 | $360.50 | $474.34 | 108.25 |
| HydroGize Water Bottle - White (15 fl oz capacity) | 5777 | $360.50 | $474.34 | 108.25 |
| Premium Shaker Bottle | 5219 | $20.25 | $26.64 | 0 |

| Accessories | Count | Item | WhSl | Retail | PV |
|---|---|---|---|---|---|
| 10 Oil Case (Blue) | 1 | 5280 | $16.25 | $21.38 | 0 |
| 10 Oil Case (Green) | 1 | 5281 | $16.25 | $21.38 | 0 |
| 10 Oil Case (Fuchsia) | 1 | 5282 | $16.25 | $21.38 | 0 |
| 30 Oil Case | 1 | 5279 | $38.25 | $50.33 | 0 |
| AromaGlide Roller Fitments | 10 | 4578 | $10.00 | $13.16 | 0 |
| AromaSpinner | 1 | 21777 | $14.75 | $19.41 | 5 |
| AromaSpinner Accessory Pack | 1 | 21778 | $6.00 | $7.89 | 0 |
| Clear Vegetable Capsules | 250 | 3193 | $7.50 | $9.87 | 0 |
| Core Vitality Case (Purple) | 1 | 5160 | $14.25 | $18.75 | 0 |
| Core Vitality Case (Teal) | 1 | 5660 | $14.25 | $18.75 | 0 |
| Easy Fill Pipettes | 15 | 4927 | $4.00 | $5.26 | 0 |
| Essential Oil Bottle Organizer | 1 | 5765 | $10.25 | $13.49 | 0 |
| Essential Oil Sample Bottle | 25 ct | 3194 | $9.75 | $12.83 | 0 |
| Glass Oil Droppers | 6 ct | 3810 | $5.00 | $6.58 | 0 |
| Oil Bottle Cap Labels (312 labels) | 1 pk | 3939 | $3.00 | $3.95 | 0 |
| Premium Display Case | 1 | 5276 | $71.00 | $93.42 | 0 |
| Vitassage w/Case | 1 | 4625 | $61.50 | $80.92 | 30.75 |
| Vitassage Case Only | 1 | 4898 | $20.25 | $26.64 | 0 |

| Samples and DIY Kit | Count | Item | WhSl | Retail | PV |
|---|---|---|---|---|---|
| DIY Kit    3 crafts for 6 people | | 21861 | $59.00 | $59.00 | 0 |
| EO Sample Pack (10 each of 5 oils) | 50 | 4940 | $45.00 | $59.21 | 22.5 |
| Lavender Sample Packets | 10 ct | 4770 | $10.00 | $13.16 | 5 |
| Lemon Sample Packets | 10 ct | 4772 | $10.00 | $13.16 | 5 |
| Peppermint Sample Packets | 10 ct | 4771 | $10.00 | $13.16 | 5 |
| Peace & Calming Sample Packets | 10 ct | 4774 | $10.00 | $13.16 | 5 |
| Purification Sample Packets | 10 ct | 5009 | $10.00 | $13.16 | 5 |
| Thieves Sample Packets | 10 ct | 4773 | $10.00 | $13.16 | 5 |

# ALLERGEN PRODUCT GUIDE

## CONTAINS GLUTEN

5-Day Nutritive Cleanse
Allerzyme™
Animal Scents® Kit
Animal Scents® Ointment
Balance Complete™
Bar Soaps - All
Boswellia Wrinkle Cream™
Ecuadorian Dark Chocolessence™
Einkorn Products
Essentialzymes-4™
ICP™
JuvaPower™
KidScents MightyVites™
Master Formula™
MultiGreens™
Wolfberry Crisp Chocolate Bars™

## CONTAINS WHEAT GERM OIL

Animal Scents® Ointment
ART® Day Activator
ART® Night Reconstructor
Genesis Hand and Body Lotion
KidScents Bath Gel
KidScents Lotion
KidScents Shampoo
KidScents Tender Tush
Lavender Foaming Hand Soap
Lavender Volume Shampoo
Lavender Volume Conditioner
Massage Oil - Cel-Lite Magic™
Massage Oil - Dragon Time™
Massage Oil - Ortho Ease®
Massage Oil - Ortho Sport®
Massage Oil - Relaxation™
Massage Oil - Sensation™
Orange Blossom Facial Wash
Prenolone Plus™
Protec™
Regenolone™ Moisturizing Cream
Sensation Hand and Body Lotion
V-6 Advanced Vegetable Oil Complex™
Wolfberry Eye Cream™

## CONTAINS WHOLE NUTS

Gary's True Grit Einkorn Granola
Slique Bars

## CONTAINS COCONUT OIL

Essential Oils
InTouch™
KidScents™ oils - All
Oola™ oils - All
Progessence Plus™
Reconnect™
Roll-Ons - All
Valor™

Other Products
5-Day Nutritive Cleanse
Animal Scents® Dental Pet Chew
Animal Scents® Kit
Animal Scents® Shampoo
AromaGuard® Deodorants
ART® - Creme Masque
Bar Soaps - All
Bath Bombs - All
Boswellia Wrinkle Cream™
Cel-Lite Massage Oil™
Copaiba Vanilla Moisturizing Shampoo
Copaiba Vanilla Moisturizing Conditioner
Genesis Hand & Body Lotion™
KidScents® Lotion
KidScents® Slique™ Toothpaste
KidScents® Tender Tush
Lavender Mint Daily Shampoo
Lavender Mint Daily Conditioner
Lavender Volume Shampoo™
Lavender Volume Conditioner™
Lip Balm - All
Massage Oil - Dragon Time™
Massage Oil - Ortho Ease®
Massage Oil - Ortho Sport®
Massage Oil - Relaxation™
Massage Oil - Sensation™
MindWise™
Orange Blossom Facial Wash
Prenolone Plus™
Regenolone™ Moisturizing Cream
Rose Ointment™
Sensation Hand & Body Lotion™
Slique® CitraSlim™
V-6 Advanced Vegetable Oil Complex™
Wolfberry Crisp Bars
Wolfberry Eye Cream™

# ALLERGEN PRODUCT GUIDE

## CONTAINS ALMOND OIL

Essential Oils
3 Wise Men™
Acceptance™
GeneYus™
Hope™
Into the Future™
Present Time™
Reconnect™
SARA™
White Angelica™

Other Products
Bath Bombs - All
Boswellia Wrinkle Cream™
Cel-Lite Massage Oil™
Genesis Hand & Body Lotion™
KidScents® Tender Tush
Lavender Volume Shampoo™
Lavender Volume Conditioner™
Lip Balm - All
Massage Oil - All
Protec™
Sensation Hand & Body Lotion™
V-6 Advanced Vegetable Oil Complex™
Wolfberry Eye Cream™

## CONTAINS CORN

5-Day Nutritive Cleanse
AlkaLime®
Allerzyme™
AromaBright Toothpaste
Bar Soaps - All
Boswellia Wrinkle Cream™
Copaiba Vanilla Moisturizing Shampoo
Copaiba Vanilla Moisturizing Conditioner
Genesis Hand & Body Lotion™
KidScents® Lotion
KidScents® Slique® Toothpaste
KidScents® Tender Tush
Lavender Mint Daily Shampoo
Lavender Mint Daily Conditioner
Lavender Volume Shampoo™
Lavender Volume Conditioner™
Orange Blossom Facial Wash
Sensation Hand & Body Lotion™
Slique® Gum
Slique® Shake
Wolfberry Eye Cream™

## CONTAINS SOY

5-Day Nutritive Cleanse
Animal Scents® Kit
Animal Scents® Ointment
AromaGuard® Deodorants
ART® - Creme Masque
Bar Soaps - All
Copaiba Vanilla Moisturizing Shampoo
Copaiba Vanilla Moisturizing Conditioner
Genesis Hand & Body Lotion™
KidScents® Lotion
KidScents® Slique™ Toothpaste
KidScents® Tender Tush
Lavender Mint Daily Shampoo
Lavender Mint Daily Conditioner
Lavender Volume Shampoo™
Lavender Volume Conditioner™
Orange Blossom Facial Wash
Prenolone Plus™
Regenolone™ Moisturizing Cream
Rose Ointment™
Sensation Hand & Body Lotion™

## CONTAINS DAIRY

5-Day Nutritive Cleanse
Allerzyme™
Balance Complete™
Pure Protein Complete™
Super C Chewables

## NOT VEGAN

5-Day Nutritive Cleanse
Allerzyme™
BLM™
Inner Defense™
Lavender Volume Shampoo™
Lavender Volume Conditioner™
Lip Balm - All
Longevity™
Master Formula™
MultiGreens™
OmegaGize™
Prostate Health™
Pure Protein Complete™
Slique® Bars
Super C™
Super Cal Plus™
Thyromin™

# HEALTHY LIFESTYLE ANALYSIS

## INSTRUCTIONS

Take the test by truthfully answering the questions about your lifestyle. There are ten areas that will be covered: exercise, sleep, water intake, fruit and veggies, medications, coffee, alcohol, cigarettes, soda and filler drinks, and your weight. Each answer has a total points value. Once you circle each answer, check the point value for that answer at the top of the chart and write your points in each box to the right of the question. Add up all the boxes for your total score at the bottom, then check how you are doing on the Health Analysis.

## HEALTH ANALYSIS

*80-100 POINTS:* You're doing great! Keep up the good work! Did you know that your body is the perfect foundation for essential oils to work effectively and quickly? The alkaline environment that you are working so hard to maintain helps essential oils do their job whenever you use them. Continue to use essential oils in your daily regimen to maintain health and wellness.

*65-79 POINTS:* You're alright but could use some improvement in some areas. Consider looking at one or two areas that you scored low on, and work at bringing those numbers up. You can do it! Your body will thank you for it! Essential oils work well on and in your body, but they have to do some extra work to clean up a bit before they can truly be effective. You might consider taking AlkaLime™ to increase the alkaline content in your body.

*50-64 POINTS:* Your mind and body needs you to up your game! While you have a good handle on several things, you are poorly lacking in other areas. Take one item per month and work to improve your score. Retake the test each month until you start to feel better. Essential oils will help you with any emotional stress and specific topical support. Be mindful of drinking more water and add some supplements to support your health such as AlkaLime™ to help support a more alkaline environment and Thyromin™ to help support your metabolism and energy levels.*

*10-49 POINTS:* My friend, you have a lot of work to do. Essential oils will help you, but in ways that may not be expected. There will be a high level of detox in your body as essential oils work to help eliminate toxins from your body. Normal and common oil responses for others, such as calming and emotional support, may work the opposite for you by wiring you and causing detox symptoms in the form of headaches and rashes. The oils are doing their job, but it is important that you do your job, too! Consider drastically improving your health by taking some big steps toward healing through diet, exercise, and lifestyle changes. Take a look at the many supplements Young Living offers to help specific targeted areas of your life. Talk to the person who shared this test with you, and use them as your health advocate and accountability partner. They would be thrilled to help you toward a more vitality-filled life!

*\*These statements have not been evaluated by the Food and Drug Administration. These statements are not intended to diagnose, cure, treat, or prevent any disease.*

POINT VALUE PER COLUMN:

| 10 | 9 | 8 | 7 | 6 | 5 | 4 | 3 | 2 | 1 |
|----|---|---|---|---|---|---|---|---|---|

### HOW OFTEN DO YOU EXERCISE PER WEEK?
30 or more minutes per day is considered healthful.

| 10 | 9 | 8 | 7 | 6 | 5 | 4 | 3 | 2 | 1 | POINTS |
|----|---|---|---|---|---|---|---|---|---|--------|
| 7x+ | 6x | 5x | 4x | 3x | 2x | 1x | | | 0x | |

### HOW MANY HOURS OF SLEEP DO YOU GET PER NIGHT?
The average adult needs 8-9 hours per night.

| 10 | 9 | 8 | 7 | 6 | 5 | 4 | 3 | 2 | 1 | POINTS |
|----|---|---|---|---|---|---|---|---|---|--------|
| 9 | | 8 | 7 | | 6 | 5 | 4 | 3 | | |

### HOW MANY OUNCES OF WATER DO YOU DRINK PER DAY?
A gallon per day for most adults is correct if you exercise. 175lb adult = 96-128oz.

| 10 | 9 | 8 | 7 | 6 | 5 | 4 | 3 | 2 | 1 | POINTS |
|----|---|---|---|---|---|---|---|---|---|--------|
| 128oz+ | 112oz | 96oz | 80oz | 64oz | 48oz | 32oz | 16oz | 8oz | 0oz | |

### HOW MANY SERVINGS OF FRUITS & VEGGIES DO YOU EAT PER DAY?
A total of 13-15 servings per day is best. 1 serving = 1 cup or the size of your fist.

| 10 | 9 | 8 | 7 | 6 | 5 | 4 | 3 | 2 | 1 | POINTS |
|----|---|---|---|---|---|---|---|---|---|--------|
| 15+ | 13 | 10 | 8 | 5 | 4 | 3 | 2 | 1 | 0 | |

### HOW MANY PRESCRIPTION MEDICATIONS ARE YOU ON?
Prescription medications are highly acidic in most cases. Consult your doctor.

| 10 | 9 | 8 | 7 | 6 | 5 | 4 | 3 | 2 | 1 | POINTS |
|----|---|---|---|---|---|---|---|---|---|--------|
| 0 | | 1 | | 2 | | 3 | | 4 | 5+ | |

### HOW MANY CUPS OF COFFEE DO YOU DRINK PER DAY?
Coffee is highly acidic and lowers your immunity.

| 10 | 9 | 8 | 7 | 6 | 5 | 4 | 3 | 2 | 1 | POINTS |
|----|---|---|---|---|---|---|---|---|---|--------|
| 0 | | | 1 | | 2 | | 3 | | 4+ | |

### HOW MANY ALCOHOLIC BEVERAGES DO YOU DRINK PER WEEK?
Alcohol is loaded with processed sugar and is highly acidic.

| 10 | 9 | 8 | 7 | 6 | 5 | 4 | 3 | 2 | 1 | POINTS |
|----|---|---|---|---|---|---|---|---|---|--------|
| 0 | 1 | 2 | 3 | 4 | 5 | 6 | 7 | 8+ | | |

### HOW MANY PACKS OF CIGARETTES DO YOU SMOKE PER DAY?
Cigarettes lower your immunity.

| 10 | 9 | 8 | 7 | 6 | 5 | 4 | 3 | 2 | 1 | POINTS |
|----|---|---|---|---|---|---|---|---|---|--------|
| 0 | | | | 1 | | 2 | | 3+ | | |

### HOW MANY SODAS & FILLER DRINKS DO YOU DRINK PER DAY?
Sodas and filler drinks such as juice and teas are highly acidic and full of sugar.

| 10 | 9 | 8 | 7 | 6 | 5 | 4 | 3 | 2 | 1 | POINTS |
|----|---|---|---|---|---|---|---|---|---|--------|
| 0 | | | 1 | | 2 | | 3 | | 4+ | |

### HOW MANY POUNDS ARE YOU AWAY FROM YOUR GOAL WEIGHT?
Check online for what a healthy weight for your age and height should be.

| 10 | 9 | 8 | 7 | 6 | 5 | 4 | 3 | 2 | 1 | POINTS |
|----|---|---|---|---|---|---|---|---|---|--------|
| 0 | 5 | 10 | 15 | 20 | 25 | 30 | 35 | 40 | 45+ | |

**TOTAL POINTS**

Add up all the points boxes for your total score here, then check how you are doing on the Health Analysis.

# 128 HOT WORDS

Ever wonder, "What exactly is a hot word?" Here is a list of words that are considered non-compliant by the FDA and if you are a representative of Young Living, you may not use them when sharing about any of the products.

If you are talking about a word, such as cancer, but you are not implying or stating it treats this word, then it is OK to be used. If you wanted to discuss essential oils and seizures, that would be fine if you are discussing which oils could potentially CAUSE a seizure. In the case of allergies, you might talk about how a person may or may not be allergic to essential oils.

Note: There are more hot words than are listed here. Remember to use the rule of thumb: if the word implies or describes a disease or illness, that is not compliant.

Anal Fissure
Antibacterial
Anti-inflammatory
Antifungal
Antiviral
Abrasion
ADD Attention Deficit Disorder
ADHD Attention Deficit Hyperactivity Disorder
AIDS Acquired Immunodeficiency Syndrome
Allergies
Alzheimer's
Anorexia
Anxiety
Arthritis
Asthma
Autism
Autoimmune Disease
Bacteria
Bruise
Bug (as in cold or flu)
Bug & Insect Repellent

Bulimia
Burns
Bursitis
Cancer
Canker Sore
Carpal Tunnel Syndrome
Celiac Disease
Chronic Fatigue
Cold
Cold Sore
Congestion
Constipation
Contagion
Convulsion
COPD Chronic Obstructive Pulmonary Disease
Cough
Cramps
Crohn's Disease
Cystic Acne
Dandruff
Dementia

Depression
Dermatitis
Diabetes
Diarrhea
Disease
Disorder
Diverticulitis
Ear Ache
Eczema
Epidemic
Epilepsy
Erectile Dysfunction
Fever
Fibromyalgia
Flu
Fungus
Gallstones
GERD Gastroesophageal Reflux Disease
Germ
Gum Disease
Hashimoto's
Headache
Heart Attack
Heartburn
Hemorrhoids
Herpes
High Blood Pressure
High Cholesterol
HIV Human Immunodeficiency Virus
Hives
Hypertension
Hyperthyroidism
Hypothyroidism
IBS Irritable Bowel Syndrome
Illness
Infection
Infertility
Inflammation
Influenza
Insomnia
Kidney Stones
Lice
Lupus

Lyme Disease
Malady
Migraine
Mucus
Multiple Sclerosis
Nausea
Obesity
Osteoporosis
Pain
Panic Attack
Parasites
PCOS Polycystic Ovary Syndrome
Pink Eye or Conjunctivitis
Pneumonia
Post-Nasal Drip
Psoriasis
Rash
Restless Legs Syndrome
Rheumatic Fever
Rheumatoid Arthritis
Ringworm
Scars
Sciatica
Seizures
Sinusitis
Skin Tag
Sore
Sore Throat
STD Sexually Transmitted Disease
Strep Throat
Stroke
Syndrome
Tinnitus
Tooth Decay
Toxemia
Tumor
Ulcerative Colitis
Ulcers
Urinary Tract Infection
Varicose Vein
Vertigo
Warts
Yeast Infection

# INDEX

# INDEX

# AUTHOR BIOGRAPHY

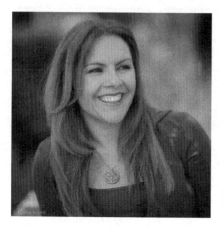

Jen O'Sullivan, a Young Living member since 2007 and Gold leader, is one of the most followed Young Living distributors because she is known for her up-front and to the point education style. She gives more free educational content on a regular basis than anyone in the Young Living industry and is the author of five Amazon best-sellers that may be purchased as a bundle pack or in bulk through 31oils.com. She, along with over 100 Young Living distributors, have developed the largest most comprehensive essential oil education and recipe usage app on the market today called "The EO Bar". She also offers an easy to use app for the Premium Starter Kit called "Live Well with Young Living". She is certified in French Medicinal Aromatherapy through The New York Institute of Aromatic Studies and has been a professional educator since 1999, at both the collegiate and high school levels. She is lovingly known as "The oil lady to the oil ladies" and has a desire to help educate anyone interested in essential oils. Her online education group of over 220,000 oil enthusiasts called "The Human Body and Essential Oils" is her main group where she teaches proper usage and safety with essential oils. She has studied health and nutrition since 2007 and has the ability to take complicated information and share it in a way that makes it easy to understand. Jen lives in Southern California with her husband Tim, who was also her high school sweetheart, and their son Jacob. Her desire is for everyone to use essential oils and learn how they can easily incorporate them into a more healthful lifestyle.

## OTHER BOOKS BY JEN

*The Essential Oil Truth: the Facts Without the Hype*
48 micro lessons to help you better understand the world of essential oils.

*French Aromatherapy: Essential Oil Recipes & Usage Guide*
The essential oil users guide to proper French method use.

*Essential Oil Make & Takes: Over 60 DIY Projects and Recipes for the Perfect Class*
DIY Make & Take projects for both beginner and intermediates.

*Essentially Driven: Young Living Essential Oils Business Handbook*
The easiest resource to help you get your YL business started the right way.

*Live Well: Essential Oils for Wellness, Purpose, and Abundance*
A full color "Oils 101" class in a book focusing on the Premium Starter Kit.